Advance Praise

"Straight talk from a straight shooter. Bob and I began as client/counsel on many Discovery Communications real estate transactions; just as those developed into a complex headquarters project, our relationship has grown into friendship. Bob's book deals with many life challenging topics like health management, child rearing, and even the possibility of miracles. You may not have the same background or experiences, but in his story Bob gives insights that will certainly make you ask 'what if?' and perhaps even influence future choices. Kudos to the Brams family for sharing this battle and continuing the fight!"

—Pandit Wright, former senior executive of Discovery Communications Inc. and president and CEO of the Boys & Girls Clubs of Greater Washington

"I have the honor and privilege of reviewing Bob Brams's new book, *Forever Optimistic*. This story of his survival against all odds is nothing short of extraordinary. Bob walks us through a harrowing tale of his two craniotomies on both the East and West Coasts as well as radiation and chemotherapy treatments. Following his first surgery, Bob battled a stroke, a coma, life support, multiple ICUs, and even hemophilia. Bob was left with difficulties walking, thinking, and speaking; and he had to undergo lengthy 24/7 care at the National Rehabilitation Hospital in Washington, DC followed by years of therapy.

In the aftermath of his myriad medical procedures, problems, and therapy, he began to search his soul on how he had led his life and what it takes to lead a successful and fulfilling life. Bob

explores many of the precise issues that have come up throughout my many years of practice. Bob's thoughts and conclusions
are spot on. Bob has a lovely wife and two children so he's seen
a lot. I found the book fascinating, captivating, and full of keen
insights about life's many trials. Brain tumor or not, I believe that
all readers from parents, to students, to professionals—virtually
anyone will find Bob's book to be a thoroughly insightful and
captivating read."

**—Jerrold M. Post, MD, professor emeritus, George
Washington University, and former president,
Political Psychology Associates, Ltd.**

"While always self-effacing, our author Bob Brams never under-
estimates himself. His new book paints a picture of man struck
down by a brain cancer diagnosis at the peak of his legal career.
He fights the battle with unrelenting courage, common sense,
humor, and proportionality. With his cancer diagnosis, he fell
from a high perch; Bob had risen to the top of the vaunted
Washington, DC legal profession. He did so through hard work
and his gift for the law. Indeed, one of the reasons that he's risen
so high is that he always asserts only well-reasoned arguments.
Bob also has an uncanny ability to never let his professional relationship with adversaries interfere with the personal relationship
he would develop with them. He has maintained friendships
with clients and adversaries to this day. Confronting a deadly
brain tumor, Bob has applied his positive attitude, force of character, and diligence to achieve a quality life of a different sort,
as he shares in this riveting account of his illness, *pas de deux* with
the medical profession, and application of his life skills to a new
normal. This is must read for a broad range of readers from

those struggling through a devastating illness or other situations to those individuals struggling to find success in law, business, and life."

**—Judge Christine O. C. Miller,
United States Court of Federal Claims (Ret.)**

"I'm honored to endorse Bob Brams's book: *Forever Optimistic.* Bob's medical experience was nothing short of devastating, but he's come out of it all with the greatest of insights on choosing your path and leading life. Bob's battle back from tragedy has led him to reflect on valuable thoughts on overcoming failures to benefiting from his many achievements in the legal profession. Bob and I go back a number of years. Bob's son Garrett and I were on competing wrestling teams and we frequently found ourselves in the same gyms. Bob's cancer battle took him right up to the edge of death. He's definitely been the beneficiary of so many miracles that only the good Lord can provide. While he fights on with continually perplexing MRIs, Bob's come out of it all with wisdom that should be invaluable for all. Bob's book is inspirational, motivational, and chock full of key lessons for leading a successful life. I'm confident that Bob's story will be powerful and healing for so many."

**—Kyle Snyder, US Olympic Wrestling gold medalist
and three-time NCAA Division I Wrestling champion**

"Robert Brams wrestled all his life, as did his son. Robert then became a top law partner in his field over the past thirty years. Most people might look at Robert Brams's situation and wonder how anyone could remain optimistic when faced with the challenges that have confronted him and still haunt him today.

Through multiple hospital stays, setback after setback, and a litany of medical complexities, the journey outlined in *Forever Optimistic* has been nothing short of extraordinary. Bob's story is both inspirational and motivational, particularly when you consider how he's always moved forward with an optimistic eye. *Forever Optimistic* might even be underselling Robert's outlook on life. His resolve to power on, to demonstrate the best of human spirit, and to fight through it all and still stay positive has been nothing short of incredible."

—Mike Moyer, executive director of the National Wrestling Coaches Association

"Bob Brams's book, *Forever Optimistic*, takes us through his devastating experiences that remind us of both our fragility and resilience. The situation, with which he still does battle, leads us down a trail filled with inspiration and valuable insights. It is a beautiful story of individual perseverance weaved with the indispensable role of family, prayer, and love."

—DeMaurice Smith, executive director, National Football League Players Association

"What an incredible achievement and a beautiful memoir of Bob's extraordinary journey and how he has always seen the good and inspired everyone around him. I am truly moved and deeply touched. Congratulations. It makes for fascinating reading, and I am sure will be a great help for many patients."

—Dr. Henry Brem, chief of Neurosurgery, Johns Hopkins Medicine, Harvey Cushing professor of Medicine

"I so enjoyed reading through this marvelous collection of experiences and thoughts from Bob Brams on his personal journey with a brain tumor. Throughout this body of work, Bob chronicles his trials and tribulations and shows how true grit and determination can get anyone through this with the right attitude and expectations. This is a must-read by not only patients who will share the same experiences and thoughts, but also for caregivers or anyone who would appreciate what it takes to move through this process successfully. I admire Bob for taking the time to share his thoughts. I certainly learned a lot which will ultimately make me a more understanding and compassionate physician and surgeon."

—Dr. Mitchel Berger, chief of Neurosurgery, University of California San Francisco Medicine, and Blue Ribbon panelist of President Joe Biden's Moonshot Blue Ribbon Panel

"I met Bob probably fifteen years ago when he was already well into his career as a partner at the law firm of Patton Boggs. I knew from our first meeting that I would develop a good long term relationship with Bob because he is smart and ethical. He's not only a top lawyer, but he also has a great business sense. He combines these attributes with a focus on the importance of methodically achieving success in every matter assigned to him. Over the years our relationship grew about our shared passion for infrastructure and the government's role in being a catalyst to make things happen.

It is not surprising to me to see how Bob has tackled his illness, never giving up, always driving to find the right solution, and surrounding himself with family and friends to share the energy needed to be successful. I have no doubt that Bob will be successful in overcoming his current health challenge. Bob's positive attitude continues to inspire and motivate me every day."

—Frederick Werner, executive vice president, AECOM

"I am very honored that Bob Brams asked me to say a few words about his new book, *Forever Optimistic*. I got to know Bob through our mutual love of the sport of wrestling. Both of us were college wrestlers and learned the lessons the sport teaches so well; hard work, persistence, and determination. We both watched as our sons learn the same lessons from the sport. When Bob was suddenly diagnosed with brain cancer, my heart was broken for him and his family. But I knew that if anyone could beat this insidious disease, it would be Bob with his determination, his good humor, and his comments like 'Alan, I have only one thing to do. It's to win and stay here for my family and friends.' Bob's book is his story. I am so proud of him and I know that everyone that reads this will be inspired. Love you, Bob."

—Alan Meltzer, CEO, NFP/ The Meltzer Group Mid-Atlantic

"At a time in history when unsettling societal pressures have converged to create unprecedented angst and frustration, Bob's inspirational words grounded in fundamental truths are a welcome beacon along life's often difficult path to a meaningful existence. I first met Bob more than a decade ago when I served on the New Jersey attorney general's executive team and as an advisor to the governor of the Garden State. I engaged him as outside counsel to help respond to the federal government's (intentionally) high-profile and contentious demand for the return of $271 million in grant proceeds expended in connection with the cancelled ARC Tunnel public transportation connector project into New York City. Bob and his team offered invaluable expertise and calming strategic advice at a boiling point in the dispute, thereby facilitating an amicable and advantageous resolution for New Jersey.

Later, when responding to the devastating impacts unleashed by [Super Storm] Sandy in October 2012, as 'Storm Czar' I again called on Bob to counsel the State on grant processes that complied with complex federal regulations relating to vital reconstruction projects. Undeniably, he showed exceptional capabilities as a lawyer, but it was his infectious positive energy that fueled our enduring friendship. *Forever Optimistic* delivers simple, but highly poignant, wisdom through the lens of a compelling, real-world account of Bob's courage, remarkable perseverance, and accomplishments in the face of the kind of adversity that's never planned for. His engaging and accessible writing style effortlessly carries us through arduous accounts of heartache and triumph that unassumingly capture the unique and insightful spiritual person he is. He relies on genuine, thoughtful, and smart prose to provoke, but never patronize. As I turned through the pages, I found myself reevaluating who I am and what I stand for—and feeling thankful for the experience. The reader is invited into Bob's journey in vivid and unfiltered ways that necessarily inspire deep introspection and frankness with oneself. He unselfishly shares intimate moments as a backdrop to deliver life lessons, while empowering us to reexamine our reasons for being. Indeed, the book motivates us to be better human beings—better spouses, better parents, better friends, better neighbors, and better co-workers. If living life to the fullest is important to you, *Forever Optimistic* is a must read in 2021."

—Marc-Philip Ferzan, management advisory services firm leader; former government executive and cabinet-level advisor

FOREVER OPTIMISTIC

FOREVER OPTIMISTIC

Fighting Brain Cancer, Finding
Your Best Path, and Leading a
Life With Purpose

Robert S. Brams

WITH A FOREWORD BY UNITED
STATES SENATOR CHRIS COONS

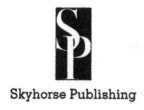

Skyhorse Publishing

Skyhorse Publishing books may be purchased in bulk at special discounts for sales promotion, corporate gifts, fundraising, or educational purposes. Special editions can also be created to specifications. For details, contact the Special Sales Department, Skyhorse Publishing, 307 West 36th Street, 11th Floor, New York, NY 10018 or info@skyhorsepublishing.com.

Skyhorse® and Skyhorse Publishing® are registered trademarks of Skyhorse Publishing, Inc.®, a Delaware corporation.

Visit our website at www.skyhorsepublishing.com.

10 9 8 7 6 5 4 3 2 1

Library of Congress Cataloging-in-Publication Data is available on file.

Cover design by Kai Texel

Print ISBN: 978-1-5107-6616-7
Ebook ISBN: 978-1-5107-6617-4

Printed in the United States of America

Dedication

This book is dedicated to my mother, Renee Brams, who passed away on March 30, 2020. Mom, you are forever in my heart, my soul, and my mind. Your support on this book prior to your passing was invaluable. The lessons you've taught me throughout life will live on forever. You and Dad taught me well! I'm confident you'll read a final copy of this book one day and you'll give me more valuable edits. I love you, Mom and Dad.

Author's Note

After outlining in this book my near-death medical experience, I set about one of my primary purposes for this writing—to be incredibly positive about all we can do in all aspects of life! I want to pass on what I've learned over many years, a host of experiences, and the perspective I've developed by going through and continuing to fight the brain cancer battle.

My goal is to inspire students, parents, business people, and the like to really explore their passions and interests in life and to set along a path to achieve meaningful objectives. I know finding your passion is no easy task and requires that you follow different paths and that you engage in some thoughtful introspection. While the practice of law was my passion for over thirty years, my medical plight has caused me to pursue a new critical passion: to help find a cure for brain cancer.

The important role you can fill: Please consider joining our "fight brain cancer" team by making a donation or by otherwise supporting our efforts. We will be pursuing our efforts along with some of the finest neurosurgery and neuro-oncology teams and medical institutions in the world, namely Johns Hopkins Medicine, the University of California San Francisco, and Oligo Nation, a non-profit focused on fighting a rare brain tumor called an oligodendroglioma, the precise type of tumor that affects me and many others throughout the world. Fortunately, my relationships with the Biden Administration and some of the top public policy firms in the country will allow our cancer fight to be heard at the highest of levels. Sadly, President Biden's son Beau passed away from brain cancer, so Biden's Moonshot Initiative to fight brain cancer takes on even greater significance.

Let's Fight Together to Beat Brain Cancer. Please consider being part of the team by donating at the following website:

1MBBC.com

Donors and other contributors are recognized on the website.

Table of Contents

Foreword

By United States Senator Chris Coons

I am honored to prepare this foreword for Bob Brams's new book: *Forever Optimistic: Fighting Brain Cancer, Finding Your Best Path, and Leading a Life with Purpose.*

Bob and I went to neighboring and competing high schools in Wilmington, Delaware, where, among other things, we were both involved in the sport of wrestling—a definite character builder for life! We went our separate ways after high school, and we both ended up becoming lawyers.

We met again years later in Washington, DC, at a fund raiser hosted in my honor at Bob's law firm, Patton Boggs. The event was held before my first Senate term, and I met Bob along with his partner, the late, venerable Tommy Boggs. It was great seeing Bob, another Delawarean working in Washington, DC.

Bob and I crossed paths again in the last couple years at two major wrestling tournaments in Delaware. We both presented at programs at those tournaments focused on the fight against cancer. Though an excellent lawyer, Bob's thirty-year law career was cut short in 2015 by a brain cancer diagnosis. Bob participated on our panels as a brain cancer survivor and former Delaware wrestler. Indeed, he has quite an inspiring story to tell.

Bob had his first brain surgery in January 2015. Just hours after surgery, his condition took a sharp turn for the worse and Bob ended up on the brink of death. He had a hemorrhagic stroke, suffered a coma, and ended up on life support. His insurers found that he had suffered a "catastrophic loss." His medical team described him as the sickest man on the neuro-intensive care unit. After years of rehabilitation and regular MRIs, Bob had to undergo a second brain surgery in 2019 to address further tumor growth.

The book runs through the harrowing details of Bob's near-death experience. Following all of his treatments and now no longer practicing law, Bob has had the time to reflect on his life, the path he chose, and how he and his wife have raised a beautiful family, their two children now both college graduates. His book focuses on what has worked and what hasn't worked for him in business and life. Above all else, Bob's story is inspirational and focuses on the importance of finding one's passion and seeing its value in helping one find success and true happiness in life.

I know the cancer battle personally as it has affected my family directly, as well as many friends. I can empathize with the struggles that Bob and his family have undergone and still go through. While I've spoken on the fight against cancer, Bob takes it a step further by writing *Forever Optimistic*. Bob's positive attitude exudes from each chapter over his long road to recovery.

Bob's story is inspiring on many levels. His story is deeply moving, surprisingly humorous, and brimming with hard won wisdom for readers from every walk of life. I hope you find deep value in reading about Bob's compelling journey.

PART ONE:

My Toughest
Match Ever

Chapter One

A Fender Bender on Willard Avenue

On a sunny afternoon in mid-December 2014, I drove through the Maryland suburbs of Washington, DC on my way to a routine cardiologist appointment.

As I approached the District of Columbia line, I stopped on Willard Avenue, intending to take a left turn onto North Park Avenue—a little shortcut to my doctor's office.

Just then a car hit mine from behind. The whiplash rocked me sharply backward, and my head and neck slammed against the headrest.

Too minor to require a police response, the accident appeared to be just one of those trifling annoyances that litter modern life. I pulled into a parking lot at the side of the road; the other driver followed me. Emerging from her car, the pleasant-looking woman asked if I was okay, and we quickly assessed the damage to the vehicles. Both cars remained drivable.

"It's so good that none of us got hurt," the woman said in a warm and friendly tone. I recall the woman appeared almost "angelic." At least, that was the first word that floated through my mind. We exchanged insurance information and went our separate ways. I never saw the woman again, and the incident did not even cause me to miss my doctor's appointment.

Fate moves in mysterious ways. At that moment I resembled most people who are caught up in normal everyday situations—I had my family (my son, daughter, and wife), schools, errands, work—the agreeable tempo of the ordinary. I didn't pay more than occasional attention to the larger questions in life. But with that unremarkable fender bender, I passed over an invisible line, the one separating "before" and "after."

Of course, I didn't realize anything of the sort at the time. We were planning on leaving for a family vacation in Mexico the next week, celebrating the holiday season with a getaway. Most of my thoughts of the future centered around clearing my work decks and getting away for winter break.

Life is what happens while you're busy making other plans. We've all heard that line often enough—John Lennon used it in a song lyric, and the sentiment goes back decades before that. Heavyweight boxing champion Mike Tyson would put it more bluntly: "Everybody has a plan, until they get punched in the mouth."

Whichever way you want to express it, I've come to embrace the idea wholeheartedly. I think of myself—the "before" Bob Brams—and I feel badly for him, for the poor guy's innocence in the face of the world of trouble that was about to come crashing down on him.

That evening, I still felt minor effects from the fender bender. I had tingling sensations in my arms and neck, pain so slight I hesitated to give it any name beyond "discomfort." I went to an Urgent Care medical facility to get checked out. The examining physician ordered an X-ray and found no broken bones. My complaint seemed to summon up a typical take-two-aspirin-and-call-me-in-the-morning response (though nowadays, it's more likely Tylenol and skip the phone call). I should consider some massage work or physical therapy, the urgent care physician suggested.

I took my tingling limbs home and dove back into clearing up my work and preparing for vacation. Life went on happening, and I went on making other plans. But the sore neck refused to go away.

I was fifty-five years old when the accident occurred. Like many couples, my loving wife Kim and I continued to be "battle tested" in raising children. As of my sixty-first birthday, we hadn't won the war yet, but as Garrett and Taylor are now both well on their way to making the transition from college to graduate schools or a career, we seem to have come through as reasonably good parents. By no means are we experts at child rearing, but we appreciate more than ever that properly raising the next generation may be one of the most important things we do in our lives.

Kim and I discussed my troublesome soreness, a minor ailment that was persisting longer than we expected.

"Why don't we call Ron?" Kim asked.

Dr. Ron Bortnick is Kim's uncle. It's always a good thing to have an in-law (that's a convenient catch-all term) who is a physician. More to the point in my case, Ron is a neurosurgeon, retired but the former head of neurosurgery at Fairfax Hospital in Virginia.

I laid out my symptoms to Ron, feeling like I must be over thinking it. "It's probably nothing," I hurried to say. "Somewhere in the midst of all that whiplash, maybe I have some bruising, that's all." That was my vaguely embarrassed thought.

"How long has it been since the accident?" Ron asked.

"What is it now? Three days?"

"I would say get an MRI, just to make sure there's nothing more serious than a little bruising going on."

"We're going on vacation," I responded. "Let's get this done now."

So I did. Generally, I have a "do it" or "let's get it done" type of personality. I tend not to waver and second-guess. Having an MRI while we were in Mexico on vacation didn't seem to be the way to go. The only reasonable thing to do was to have the procedure before we left—yep, get it done.

But life was happening and I was going to have to fit the brain scan into my busy day. I'm a lawyer, and my law partner and I were scheduled to take one of our co-workers out for lunch. And that evening, Kim and I were hosting a family holiday party at our home.

I chose Sibley Memorial Hospital in the Palisades neighborhood of Washington, DC, not due to a referral from Ron or for any specific reputation of the facility, but simply because it was located conveniently on my way home. Sibley is also owned and operated by Johns Hopkins Medicine. Between lunch with my work friends and the party with my extended family, I'd dash over, expose myself to some magnetic resonance imaging, and get to the party on time.

It was not to be.

Chapter Two
The Journey and the Struggle

I realize it's a big ask to suggest that anyone should care about another person's problems, or at least care enough to read a detailed account of them. A cynic's view: "Tragedy is when I cut my finger," said the comic Mel Brooks. "Comedy is when you fall into an open sewer and die." Fortunately, I will say I do see much more sympathy and empathy in the world when facing a serious problem.

I'm not up for challenging human nature. But my experience is made up of so much more than a blow-by-blow tally of hospital rooms, surgeons' scalpels, and heroic caregivers.

Joseph Campbell, the recognized expert on humanity's myths and legends, talks about the hero's journey in *The Hero with a Thousand Faces*. Some aspects of that mythological journey seem to hold true throughout all cultures worldwide. Again and again, the tale has similar elements. The hero ventures forth on a quest, enters a place of "darkness" and "danger," and returns with wisdom that helps the whole community.

That's what I want to do here. I'm no classical hero in the spirit of Aeneas or Ulysses, but I possess hard-earned knowledge that has come to me via a terrible struggle. I have indeed entered a place of darkness and danger, from which I emerged a changed individual. Now I want to share what I've learned in order to help others.

Through my experience, I've found the need to start thinking more critically about how my life has developed, and how I should proceed going forward, raising my family, and dealing with serious issues. My medical situation has helped to focus my attention on what I believe is important, and my thoughts revolve around a new set of the uncertainties that have now become very vivid. Hopefully my new-found perspective can help you in thinking about your own life, especially in times of pain, suffering, and uncertainty. I do feel a compulsion to write because I find it therapeutic and cathartic.

This book provides a number of thoughts on how to conduct oneself in life, with family, friends, and in business. We all hope that our children appreciate that leading lives of character and integrity will give them the greatest chance of achieving happy and fulfilling lives. I stress the importance of pursuing a career for which one has passion, which I realize is far easier said than done. How to convey these truths?

I frequently took a path in life and business that was far more arduous than it needed to be. Nevertheless, I feel fortunate to have succeeded because I developed, over time, an increasing desire to succeed. Growing up, I recall Mom saying, "Success breeds success." She was right. My failures were no fun at all, but they never really discouraged me. To the contrary, missteps always inspired me to try to figure out what went wrong and how to fix them.

I sometimes feel as though I'm racing against the clock. I

want to leave a legacy of value. I've been fortunate to have practiced law around the world for over thirty years, though health issues have forced me into an early retirement. Maybe it could prove as something of a blessing that my time is now freed up to think more carefully about life and about guiding my children.

My focus has sharpened over the last several years as to what my children need to know and do in order to succeed and be productive citizens in the world. Of course, my goal is for them to have loving and responsible relationships, to properly raise their own children, and to guide others to succeed. Fortunately, I've now had several years to think things through.

Developing the attributes to succeed in life doesn't come easily. They often must be learned and are frequently the result of finding the right experiences and avoiding the wrong ones. Sometimes you just have to make your own luck, try to position yourself to be in the right place at the right time, and appreciate that the evolution of finding your passion, particularly one that "pays the rent" isn't easy.

The trouble with the hero's journey is that it asks so much of us. Why can't we just get to the heart of things more quickly? "Couldn't I just skip that business about venturing into a place of darkness and danger? I want to go directly to the wisdom part of things!"

Getting banged up a bit is unavoidable as one seeks to determine the best choices in life. "Live and learn" is the old expression. I'm hoping this book can help minimize some of the struggles with life's steep learning curves that most of us seem to face.

This is not intended to be a depressing story. Rather, I see it as a tale of challenges, hope, and triumph, focusing on all we can do in life with the right positive attitude. Whatever difficulties you encounter, you will be amazed how much you can achieve.

My story is one of finding inspiration, passion, and optimism! Sure, I have a brain tumor, but I still feel as though I've won. As Nicole Reed said in her book *Ruining You*: "Sometimes the bad things that happen in our lives put us directly on the path to the best things that will ever happen to us."

I don't want to suggest that I'm the model for figuring out one's passion. It took me quite a while to figure things out, and I definitely had to wander (or maybe stumble) down various paths to ultimately achieve success.

Chapter Three
Keep an Eye out for Miracles

As of 2020 I have had countless encounters with MRI machines, to the point where I normally fall asleep during the noisy, claustrophobic procedure. The MRI I had at Sibley Hospital shortly after the accident was not quite so soporific, but I recall at least closing my eyes and Zen-ing out a bit.

Before the results came in, I did what one does in a hospital waiting room, which is to wait, browse through magazines, and take in a little TV. My mind was almost totally taken up with thinking about the upcoming family party that was set to begin in just a few hours. I had a mental to-do list that I went over repeatedly. If I spared any attention for the medical procedure I had just undergone, it was to speculate on just what minimal degree of trauma led to my symptoms of nerve tingling and neck pain. My expectation was firm; I was convinced that if any damage from the fender bender showed at all, it would be minor.

The radiologist trained in reading MRI results approached. He appeared concerned. "We've found a small spot on your brain," he said. He implied that the spot might be a tumor.

"What?" I asked in disbelief. I remember my thoughts tumbling one after another. *What the heck? You weren't looking for spots! You were supposed to find some swelling, maybe! At worst, I was hoping you'd find only some bruising or inflammation.* But a tumor? I never imagined that. The doctors were surprised that I was asymptomatic.

"Perhaps you had a seizure," the doctor said. "That might be what led you to have your traffic accident."

I knew very well what had happened out there on Willard Avenue. I didn't have a seizure and go off the road. Nothing like that occurred. I was stopped, totally stationary, and ready to make a turn. But I didn't say anything to challenge the seizure theory. The doctor told me they would like to hold me overnight at Sibley. They would give me some anti-seizure meds, he said.

None of this made sense to me. I knew I hadn't had a seizure, and if I hadn't had a seizure, why would my doctors prescribe anti-seizure medication? Of course, they saw it as a preventive measure, to stop a seizure from occurring.

When a situation turns surreal, the human mind tends to turn frantic, repeatedly butting its head against a stone wall, trying to figure out the inexplicable. My thoughts raced. I couldn't fully grasp what was happening. I certainly didn't conclude that I had begun a shattering journey that would transform my life. But without quite realizing it yet, I had fallen down the rabbit hole.

To the outside world, though, I presented a calm exterior.

I called Kim. "Well, they say they found a spot on my brain."

"What does that mean?" She sounded just a bit panicked.

"I don't know what it means yet. Just go ahead with the party. You don't have to come down here. It's all right."

I could almost see Kim rolling her eyes over my attempt at

stoicism. "I'll come," Kim said. She left our own ongoing party and quickly headed to Sibley.

It would turn out that the neck pain I felt after the Willard Avenue accident had nothing to do with the "spot." I was asymptomatic as far as the tumor was concerned. The pain and soreness that led me into the sleek, high-tech tunnel of the MRI proved to be simply a response to the whiplash I had experienced. It had no connection to what the MRI turned up in my brain.

Waiting for Kim, I tried to puzzle out the implications of what had just happened to me. I couldn't grasp any of it. So the traffic accident that led to the discovery of the spot on my brain was just a coincidence? Without my car being bumped from behind I would have moved ahead with my life, making plans, caught up in the day-to-day. Could all of it really be possible?

If that was the case, it went way beyond coincidence. Sitting there in the Sibley waiting room with my life upended, I remembered the calming and reassuring face of the woman who had crashed her car into mine. Again, the word "angelic" entered my mind. The woman was my guardian angel without her knowing it. Or maybe she *had* known it.

A chain of events that began on Willard Avenue had led me to Sibley Hospital a few days later. I didn't know if I believed in fate or divine intervention. My emotions were at that moment too mixed up to wrestle with such universal questions. I simply knew that I had begun a new phase of my life.

Keep an eye out for miracles, I told myself, a line that would become something of a mantra for me. This would be the first scrap of wisdom that came my way. It was just a hint of greater riches. The simple six-word sentiment rose like a blip on a radar screen and then vanished amid the tumble of my racing thoughts.

I already understood that up ahead on the hero's journey, a dark and dangerous cave was waiting for me. I didn't think about it in those terms, but I certainly knew that I might be visiting some version of hell, from which I might never emerge.

The experience, when it came, would prove awful beyond measure. I would soon earn something like a booby prize, or like a newly minted Olympic-style medal, when a group of physicians described me as "the sickest person on the ward." The ward they were referring to was the neuro intensive care unit at Johns Hopkins Medicine. That's where I would face the greatest challenge of my life.

Chapter Four
Unraveling the Medical Questions

I ultimately learned that the type of tumor I have is called an oligodendroglioma. Surprising to me, in this day and age, was the fact that the doctors really could not definitively identify the true status of the tumor without cutting my head open. Was it static, slow-growing, or fast-growing? From a medical perspective, the brain can be quite unpredictable, and a lot still remains to be discovered.

I would later hear a brain surgeon suggest that after the passage of time, "the cells can get a little angrier." A slow-growing tumor could develop into a faster-growing tumor without any clear explanation, other than a newly active division of cells. It all demonstrated the unfathomable nature of the brain.

The radiologists at Sibley said that the small area they detected showed a relatively small tumor: Ten millimeters, less than half an inch, or the length of a thumbnail. Sibley was an excellent hospital, and the staff there were experts. Of course, I could take their analysis as gospel, right?

That wasn't the way I approached things. In my more than thirty years in the legal world, I learned to question everything, especially the views of so-called experts. So I didn't accept the first opinion, or even the second or third. I had my MRIs reviewed by the top doctors in various major medical centers around the country, including Georgetown University Medical Center, George Washington University Medical Center, Duke University Medical Center, Sloan Kettering, and Harvard.

An MRI scan is merely shadows on a sheet of film. They mean nothing until they are examined by trained specialists who have spent their lives learning how to read the shadows and translate them into real-world results.

Networking proved to be a vital part of the medical process. Under the circumstances, Kim and I happened to have the perfect neighbor. A lot of people in this alienated society don't even know their neighbors, but I knew ours. That was one more case where I was lucky to possess a friendly and open personality. It proved crucial. While my MRIs were going out to the best hospitals in the country, I reached out to a friend from just down the street, Dr. Jeff Jacobson, a top neurosurgeon at Johns Hopkins at the time (and now at Georgetown University Hospital).

Jeff offered to look at my MRI one Friday evening. Not exactly your typical pre-weekend get-together for cocktails and appetizers, because it would include an informal analysis of my scans. Professional, with a calming personality, the good doctor brought his prodigious experience to bear on my MRI. It was a cold evening that became even colder when he confirmed our worst fears.

"This isn't a very small, ten-millimeter tumor," he said quietly, dismissing the optimistic opinions of another physician. "To the contrary, I'm convinced that you have quite a large, six-centimeter-by-three-centimeter tumor in your brain."

Not a thumbnail, in other words, but more like the size of a golf ball. I did the math late in the writing process, and frankly, it still makes me feel uncomfortable. The tumor turned out to be ten times the size of what the doctors had originally estimated.

Jeff immediately emailed his friend at Johns Hopkins, Dr. Henry Brem. At no time was Jeff exuding confidence over the prospects of an easy road for me. In hindsight, perhaps I should have been a little frightened that Jeff didn't offer to take the case himself, as he's done plenty of brain surgeries over his long and successful career. I prefer to just look at it as the etiquette of a good neighbor. Perhaps knowing the person on whom you operate interferes with objectivity.

It may sound like overkill—the multiple MRI reviews from specialists nationwide, plus consultation with neighbors, network contacts, and friends of friends. But I felt that I had no choice. While one hospital was telling me that I had only a very small, ten-millimeter tumor, another emergency room sent me away one day telling me that it might be nothing. However, the next day, that same hospital gave me an MRI report that identified a tumor that was far larger than originally estimated.

To add to my confusion and distress, many years before, when I was experiencing some headaches, my internist recommended that I have an MRI. At that time, several highly qualified doctors reviewed the results. They characterized what they saw in my brain as simply scar tissue. They concluded that the scar tissue needed no further review. However, other neurosurgeons were telling me in 2015 that they might have investigated further based on my MRI of many years earlier!

Even apart from the sizable mass on my brain, my head was spinning with uncertainty from all the different views by different radiologists and neurosurgeons that were among the best in the world.

As an attorney, it had always been my practice to question even the best of authorities. I believe the best option is to always "trust your gut." I never give up on common sense, even in areas where I have virtually no knowledge and certainly no training.

Ultimately, the consensus appeared to be that I would need a craniotomy to have the tumor surgically removed. The term "craniotomy" was a new one for me, or at least it was never a term that had ever popped up in a sentence referring to my very own cranium. Concerning, yes, and more than that, pretty damn frightening.

At that point, worries were being stacked upon worries, but I felt the healthiest thing to do was not to panic. I don't intend to sound too brave, but I believe that my energy is better spent on finding the best solution to any problem. It was absolutely essential to look at the new situation as another challenge, another opponent to beat. Instead of falling into a despairing frame of mind, I always try to respond to difficulties with a determined attitude—not "why me?" but rather "give it your best shot!" These were thinking skills that I had adopted from a long history of participation in sports during my younger years. They were further developed and strengthened in my law practice.

Although brain cancer would clearly be the biggest challenge I had ever faced, I was not facing it alone. My parents, my wife, children, other family members, and friends also had to contend with the new and very difficult development. The problem was, at that precise point in time, several of my nearest and dearest were hit with crises of their own.

Chapter Five

The Whole Family Takes a Medical Hit

In early December 2014 (before I learned of my tumor), on the evening before my son Garrett would participate in a high school wrestling tournament, I had to take him to Georgetown Hospital's emergency room. An injury he suffered at practice required stitches on his head. According to the team trainer, Garrett couldn't wrestle in the tournament the next day without written consent from an outside physician. The doctor stitched Garrett up and gave him the blessing to wrestle the next morning.

My son entered the tournament looking like a mummy, with his head wrapped in gauze bandages. He was wrestling well that day, even pinning a National Prep School All-American. However, in the midst of winning a later match, his tournament came to an abrupt halt. He heard a sickening click and felt a sharp pain. His kneecap had dislocated, literally rotating to the side of his knee.

We found ourselves back at Georgetown Hospital to see a knee surgeon. He recommended that Garrett immobilize his knee in a brace and stop wrestling completely for six weeks. That came as a big disappointment for a young man in his senior year of high school, serving as team captain, after competing without serious injury for the past dozen years.

Wrestling had become part of the Brams DNA. It was the real thing, not the entertainment version that was less a sport and more of a spectacle. I wrestled during my own youth and continued to participate in the sport as a coach, supporter, and fan.

Wrestling does great things for your mindset, but the sport is really something of a "love-hate" relationship. While you're out there on the mat in the third period, you can't imagine feeling much worse in terms of strength and lung capacity. And that's the time you really need to dig the deepest and keep pushing. And it couldn't feel worse to lose a match. On the other hand, nothing feels better than a hard-fought victory. Olympic gold medalist Dan Gable put it this way: "Once you've wrestled, everything else in life is easy."

In a wrestling match, it's just you and your opponent. You're either going to walk away on top of the world, as a winner, or with your head down, as a loser. As a middle school, high school, and college wrestler myself (in the Lehigh Valley area of Pennsylvania), and later on, watching my son compete, I came to understand that competing in wrestling naturally triggers anxiety throughout the day before your match.

I saw that kids who were too small for football or basketball naturally tended to gravitate to the wrestling mat. Wrestling is a *one on one* contest which reveals the limits of strength, smarts, agility, and quickness. Also, and perhaps more importantly, it serves as a litmus test of one's mental toughness and character.

In a tough match, you really have to dig deep to prevail. I feel like the lessons I learned from the sport were ones I have applied throughout my entire life.

So as of December 2014, Kim and I already had one child hobbling around on crutches. As if we needed more bad news, also in early December, a thyroid specialist at Children's Hospital in Washington, DC diagnosed my daughter, Taylor, with something called Graves Disease, also known as hyperthyroidism. Surgery was scheduled for Taylor in early January. But after my December traffic collision revealed my tumor, I bumped Taylor from her position in the Brams family's surgery line.

Needless to say, we canceled the Mexico vacation we had planned. On the bright side, we did have trip insurance. But the cascade of crises didn't end there.

Just as I was learning of my own health challenges in late December 2014, my then eighty-six-year-old father was feeling increasingly weak. He was having trouble caring for my mother who, for over thirty years, had been courageously living with multiple sclerosis. Sadly, Mom passed away in 2020, but she always handled her illness with great poise and very few complaints.

With my father's weakness, my parents finally decided to bring in the full-time help that they really needed. My wife, Kim, my brother, and I joined in with my parents and the caregiver to help make sure that the arrangement made sense.

My days were taken up visiting various hospitals for my own MRIs, always with the knowledge that I would soon have brain surgery. At the same time, I was ushering my father around to different hospitals, and to his own doctor, to see if anyone could figure out why he had become so weak. Given what they were going through, I felt that I couldn't tell my parents a thing about

my upcoming brain surgery. Yes, quite a dilemma on the information disclosure issue. I did inform my brother, Jon, and we
agreed that my parents didn't need the added stress.

Four days before my scheduled brain surgery, Dad's doctor
determined that a drug interaction may have been causing his
weakness. Discontinuing one of his medications, Dad began
regaining his strength. Grateful for the miraculous timing of the
improvement, we now had a brief window to share my medical news with my parents. Another miracle maybe: my father's
recovery just before my brain surgery?

Kim and I told my folks about my brain surgery, already
scheduled at Hopkins for the next week. We tried to assure them
that we didn't expect there would be any serious issues with
survival and recovery. My father is a physician himself, and my
parents were well aware that brain surgery is never easy; they
were very upset. Despite our assurances that they had nothing to
worry about, and that I would be in the hands of a top surgeon,
it turned out, as usual, they knew best.

With my father, mother, son, and daughter all afflicted with
various syndromes, injuries, or complicated health issues, Kim
was the "last (wo)man standing." I consciously tried not to wal-
low in self-pity. But the Biblical figure of Job and his myriad
troubles occurred to me more than once.

My own time in the operating room finally arrived. I tried my
damnedest to remain upbeat and optimistic. "Let's get it done,"
was my attitude. But a cruel reversal of fortune lay in wait.

Chapter Six

Brain Surgery and the Fight for My Life

"Craniotomy."

Even today, the word sends a chill down my spine. The procedure basically installs a doorway in the skull—called, inelegantly enough, a "bone flap"—through which the surgeon can enter and access brain tissue targeted for removal. Traumatic brain injury can also occasion a craniotomy, as does the installation of implants to treat Parkinson's disease, seizures, or tremors.

The brain is by far the least understood part of the human body. What is known is dwarfed by the unknown. So surgeons who enter through the craniotomy door encounter not a brightly lit, well-mapped realm, but a region rife with mystery and inexactitude.

In most cases, general anesthesia puts the patient under. But there are times where they remain awake so surgeons can gauge the effects of their work. Memorable instances include patients who continue to play the violin while on the operating table, ensuring that those areas of the brain involved in music-making remain unharmed.

In my case, Dr. Brem saw no need for me to be awake during my surgery. I was glad. The prospect of many hours under the scalpel with a hole in my head seemed none too pleasant, and I would rather be shielded from the experience via anesthesia.

Before my surgery was scheduled, I harbored a forlorn hope. Surely in this day and age a surgical team could remove a tumor with a method far less invasive than a craniotomy. Maybe, I thought, just maybe, doctors could go in through one of the other seven holes already in my head roughly in the same area as my tumor—perhaps via the ears, nose, mouth, or eyes. Maybe they could just do a biopsy for starters, or do something with lasers, or solve the problem in a far less invasive way than planned.

Even though the doctors didn't think much of my suggestions, I continued to mention options that seemed logical and less invasive to me. Experts around the country told me that my only real option was surgery to remove the tumor. If there was any positive side, they were also telling me that Johns Hopkins was the right place and Dr. Brem was the right neurosurgeon. The consistency of opinion gave me greater comfort.

As the day approached, I slipped across the line from being wholly asymptomatic and began experiencing warning signs of a brain tumor, including headaches and nausea.

As it turned out, four hours after the surgery, things went terribly wrong. My speech and responsiveness came to an abrupt halt roughly around 10:00 p.m. on the evening of my surgery. I have no recollection of the situation taking a turn for the worse. I'm told that my last few words to Kim before surgery were simple and direct.

"Keep an eye on me," I said.

Lights out. Memory out, consciousness out, and very nearly Robert Brams out.

Over the first few months of 2015, the initial conversations I had in the ICU following my surgery were the last things I recalled.

In the hours after the operation, Kim thought that I was looking particularly uncomfortable. Something just wasn't right. Kim, a clinical therapist, is very savvy and vigilant in hospital settings. Right up there with the best of them, she has an uncanny knack for staying focused on all things medical. She certainly knows when things don't appear normal. Perhaps part of it comes from having her own health problems, as well as experiencing her mother's difficult passing and her father's tragic death from a glioblastoma (better known as a GBM), another type of brain tumor. (That's right: two brain tumors in the immediate family over a fairly short time frame. As they say, aging is not for wimps).

Kim alerted the nurses at Hopkins about my symptoms late that evening. I had become very restless and nauseous. I compulsively reached for the back of my head. In her own inimitable style, Kim told the nursing staff that they needed to immediately arrange a CAT scan to see what was going on inside my head. The scan revealed that I was suffering from a cerebellum brain bleed.

To the uninitiated, a cerebellum bleed is a hemorrhagic stroke in the rear of the brain. Bleeds can indeed occur after brain surgery. But that particular one occurred on the opposite side of my head from where Dr. Brem had resected (a medical term meaning "removed") the tumor. The CAT scan result surprised both the medical team and my family. The location of the bleed did not immediately make sense.

In short order, I suffered a grand mal seizure and lost consciousness. Doctors placed me on life support. My body resembled a plumber's nightmare, with a host of tubes and drains transforming me into a swollen mess of black and blue bruises.

My condition turned critical. The medical team was unsure if I would survive this. The doctors explained to my family that any subsequent surgery to help with the bleed would likely kill me, given that I had just undergone such intrusive brain surgery. My surgeon was worried and he never appeared worried. Dr. Brem's wife described him as having the "happy gene."

I spent two weeks in the neuro intensive care unit and then two more weeks in the stroke unit. I had to be gloved and tied down so I would not inadvertently kill myself by pulling all the tubes out of my throat, head, arm, and hands. That was the point when I was nominated as "the sickest patient on the ward."

All my family could do was watch, wait, and pray. Throughout the night after my surgery, I went through multiple CAT scans. Doctors needed to monitor the bleed, anxious for signs it would stop. Of course, I was totally oblivious, but Kim and the rest of the family, as well as several of my friends, were painfully aware that my life teetered on the edge of a precipice.

Unconscious and sedated, apparently I barely responded when nurses came into my room for the next week seeking some sign of neurological reaction.

"Hey, Bob, can you wiggle your toes? Can you grip my hand? Can you open your eyes?"

After a week, the medical team took me off life support, and I continued breathing on my own. I gradually emerged from my coma, opened my eyes, and attempted to speak. Because my vocal cords had been traumatized by the intubation tube, I could manage only a feeble whisper.

I had surfaced from the realm of silence and stillness. My arms were swollen and black and blue from all the needles and IVs. I was barely functioning, but happily, I was at least orbiting the planet again.

Eventually, I had to pass a swallow test so they could avoid putting a feeding tube into me. A feeding tube is never a good thing for a host of reasons, including its tendency to introduce infection. I finally did pass the swallow test, but only after I pulled the tube out that had been inserted in my nose and down into my stomach. *Really,* I thought peevishly, *how can you expect me to swallow with a tube down my throat?*

On a cold winter night, after more than a month as a patient in the Hopkins ICU and stroke unit, I was transferred by ambulance to the National Rehabilitation Hospital (NRH) in Washington, DC. Although I don't remember much of the trip, I do recall what seemed like a long, bumpy, and cold ambulance ride that evening, wrapped up and flat on my back. I suppose I was glad to leave Hopkins, but I didn't have any say about where I would be going next for treatment.

In fact, I entered a period of total lack of control. Normally, such a situation would have bothered me immensely. But at the time I really had no independent thoughts. I had become completely dependent on my caregivers for every decision.

The NRH was my next home away from home, a third stop in a long line of hospital rooms that I hoped wouldn't stretch on forever. At NRH, I spent three-and-a-half weeks with twenty-four/seven care, receiving daily physical, occupational, and speech therapies to help me to walk, think, and speak again. I was barely functioning and pretty much out of it. I was either in a wheelchair or guided around the hallways with a belt around my waist to keep me from falling. Frankly, I barely recall the therapy.

Among the team of therapists assigned to me, I recall most vividly one therapist at NRH who seemed to feel the need to relate the awful details about the medical mess I had been through. The reason for these negativity sessions still escapes me. I really was not sure exactly why I needed to appreciate that I had just escaped from some very deep shit (Pardon my French!).

What had happened? Why did the procedure fail so spectacularly? I had lived to tell the tale. But what, exactly, was the story I had to tell? When I discovered the truth, I felt that indignity had been added to insult and injury. A crucial bit of information had slipped through the cracks, sending me hurtling right up to the edge of death.

Chapter Seven
A Catastrophic Loss and More

As they were sifting through mounds of medical records and asking very few questions, my insurance carriers labeled me "a catastrophic loss" after my surgery. Not exactly the label anyone wants. I qualified as totally disabled. I wasn't surprised. What I had been through spoke for itself. But in some ways, the quick determination made me feel that, at least statistically, I was living on borrowed time. What did those actuarial analysts in their insurance company cubicles know that I didn't? Though it sounded a bit macabre, I half-joked about having either three months or thirty years to live.

Of course, we're all living on borrowed time. No one wants to think that way. Brooding about mortality can put a little crimp in one's *joie de vivre*. Alternatively, such thoughts can prompt you to live like a bucket-list mad person, going for all the gusto you can. I ran across a quote on the internet, one of those that are attributed to Buddha but may not be anything he ever said: "The problem is, we think we have time."

I counted my blessings. I knew that life had so much to offer, and I felt extraordinarily lucky to still be around, alive and kicking (albeit just feebly kicking), able to spend my days with family and friends.

Kim, Garrett, and Taylor's love, devotion, and support couldn't have been clearer during my health crisis and the difficult months that followed. Kim, and frequently the kids, lived by my side for two months, both at Hopkins and at the National Rehabilitation Hospital.

Garrett did two things that touched me deeply. The first was a gift that he gave to himself and the whole family, which was boldly permanent. In the summer of 2015 (around five months after my surgery), he had his left bicep tattooed. At that point he was twenty years old, and I suspected he was the first in the extended family with body art. One of my earliest lessons, particularly in child-rearing, was that there are some things you just can't control. But I found it hard to complain, because the tattoo was the date of my surgery.

Second, as part of a college course, Garrett gave a very warm and touching speech about me. He sent me a video of the speech. In essence, he expressed his appreciation for all I had done for him throughout his life and how much my guidance had impacted him in a positive way. I was overcome with pride and sentiment. Like all kids, my son doesn't always listen or make sensible decisions. But his giving the speech helped affirm that as parents, perhaps Kim and I managed to do at least a few of the right things.

My daughter, Taylor, decided she wanted to investigate programs at hospitals that brought families together when facing a health crisis like ours. The idea was to allow people to share their feelings and support each other through all of the uncertainty of what are clearly difficult times. These were situations where family members were unable to speak to their loved one. They could be stuck helplessly wondering whether that person will live or die. If the patients survive, will they be able to talk, walk, and think normally? Will they be the same people that they were before surgery?

Several months after my release from NRH, it was Taylor's turn to go under the knife for the removal of her thyroid. The Brams family found itself in the middle of an odd scenario. One day I was a patient at Hopkins, and several months later I stood beside my daughter as she was about to be wheeled into the operating room at the same hospital. Perhaps we should have inquired about a family medical discount! I was proud to see that Taylor approached her surgery bravely and relieved that she recovered well.

Many valuable insights came from my experience and arose from the months-long period of mental absence from the world. Sharing my knowledge with raw honesty and even a little humor felt not only cathartic and therapeutic, but also gave me a sense of greater purpose.

Emerging from the terrible tribulations of 2015, surprisingly enough, I found myself feeling . . . happy? How was that possible? I had experienced the 1 percent complication of surgery, and came about as close to death as one could. Shouldn't I have been railing against fate like Job did? But colors seemed a little brighter, sunlight more golden, and love even more of an everyday miracle. Another quote popped up on the internet, and this one Winston Churchill really did say: "Nothing in life is so exhilarating as to be shot at without result."

I had dodged a bullet. But it turned out the battle wasn't over.

Chapter Eight

Another Challenge within the Brain

My surgery at Johns Hopkins Medicine happened on January 13, 2015. The medical team understood that, due to the almost fiendish complexity of cerebral architecture, Dr. Brem could not fully remove the brain tumor. With a glioma-type growth like I had, it is simply impossible for a surgeon to remove it all. While he could resect most of the mass, some remained. The nature of the tumor is that it's diffuse, and grows with microscopic cells, or tentacles of sorts.

The recognized strategy in such cases was to assume a "watch and wait" posture, keeping careful track of the tumor size and status via regular MRIs.

Almost four years later, on November 6, 2018, I had one of my scheduled brain scans. Ever since the surgery, they had been arranged for every two months at first, then, as long as the MRIs looked stable, every four months, then every six months. Of course, before and during each scan I prayed that my results would come back clean. Month after month, for a succession of four very anxious years, I had received good news. The tumor appeared stable.

I went into my November 2018 MRI not feeling any different than I had felt before my previous scans. Overseeing the procedure and analyzing the results was Dr. John Laterra, a co-director of the brain cancer program at Johns Hopkins Medicine. Dr. Laterra called a couple hours after my MRI, just as Kim and I were turning into our driveway.

He first asked how I was feeling. With that question, I suspected that I was about to hear some bad news.

"Unfortunately," he began—a word you definitely don't want to hear from a cancer doctor—"your scans show a very small area near the prior resection cavity that has enhanced."

"Enhanced" is a technical term that is not quite a euphemism, which describes a tumor that is growing. A region in my brain had "lit up," he said, another way to indicate the same thing. Dr. Laterra concluded that it was likely that the tumor had become more aggressive and "that it had probably gone from a Grade II to Grade III." Unfortunately, Grade III is the final grade for my tumor.

The sobering scale of brain cancers splits into "grades," according to severity. In Grade I, the tumor displays slow growth, the kind that tends not to spread into nearby tissues. These tumors may be treated without surgery, via radiation, chemotherapy, or other approaches. A Grade II tumor grows slowly, but may spread into nearby tissues or recur. That was what I had been living with for years.

Now I had apparently "graduated" to Grade III, where the tumor grows quickly, is likely to spread into nearby tissues, and displays tumor cells that look very different from normal cells. As I said, unfortunately Grade III is the final stage for a tumor such as mine, unless it evolves into a Glioblastoma Multiforme

(GBM). Development of an Oligo tumor into a GBM is a relatively rare development. A GBM is essentially unbeatable; it's the same tumor that took the lives of Senators Ted Kennedy and John McCain, as well as Beau Biden—and my father-in-law.

Quite reasonably, given the life-threatening disaster I had endured during and after my first surgery, Dr. Laterra recommended that I should not have a second surgery. Rather, he advised that I consider an aggressive course of radiation and chemotherapy in a few weeks. His thinking was simple: why do surgery when an alternative option existed—to radiate the area and do chemotherapy?

Dr. Laterra was my official "wait and see" specialist. I had come to trust him and I understood his thinking. A course of radiation and chemotherapy posed little risk of losing the patient (that would be me). Surgery, on the other hand, presented a definite risk, especially given my history.

I'm relaying this development quite calmly here, detailing cancer grades and therapy options. But of course the news of a recurrence hit me very hard. Nevertheless, I tried desperately to maintain my usual attitude of "no panic, only well-reasoned action." The words are easy enough to write on the page, but require a direct act of will to accomplish in the real world. Most of all, I dreaded giving the news to my children that the "creature" had once again awoken.

While Kim and I could well understand the "no surgery" opinion from Hopkins, we wanted to get other judgments on possible next steps. Once again, as had been the case with our neighbor, Dr. Jeff Jacobson, I happened to have a superb sympathetic resource nearby. Ashley and Alan Dabbiere resided in McLean, Virginia. Ashley, a former media executive, had recently survived surgery on the exact same rare brain tumor that I have.

A tremendously capable and energetic couple, the Dabbieres have become major advocates for brain cancer research. Partnering with the National Brain Tumor Society in 2015, a few months after my first surgery, they hosted a gala event called the Grey Soiree at their home. The fundraiser brought in over one million dollars on a night that featured a concert by the musician Sheryl Crow. While back then I still was not thinking all too clearly and was having trouble walking, I could easily grasp that the event was quite extraordinary.

My primary goal for the event was to meet and speak with Ashley Dabbiere. We quickly bonded over having the same kind of brain cancer. Oligodendrogliomas rarely occur and represent only 4 percent of all brain tumors. To have two people with the same rare tumor living just a few miles apart belied the odds. Kim and I stayed in close touch with the Dabbieres over the years as we followed each other's regular MRIs.

When the bad news arrived of a lit-up shadow on my MRI of November 2018, the Dabbieres wanted to be as helpful as possible. They suggested I contact Dr. Mitchel Berger, chief of neurosurgery at the University of California at San Francisco (UCSF), who had operated on Ashley for the resection of her oligodendroglioma. Kim and I had met Dr. Berger several times through the Dabbieres, including at Ashley's fiftieth birthday party. But we had never discussed a potential surgery with Dr. Berger.

We found ourselves getting his thoughts on the best medical course of action. We held a video conference call with Dr. Berger on November 19, 2018, during a break in a conference we were attending along with the Dabbieres. Sponsored by the National

Cancer Institute, the conference was, coincidentally and fortuitously enough, devoted to discussion of research into rare brain tumors. The event drew many of the top surgeons, scientists, and researchers from around the world, and was funded as part of the Biden "Moonshot" initiative.

Such gatherings happened periodically, but the focus of the conference in November 2018 was on, of all things, oligodendrogliomas. While it was terribly unfortunate that my tumor had enhanced, the timing could not have been better, given the type of brain tumor that was under review at the conference and the quality of the individuals at that very moment reviewing the research. I couldn't have asked to have a more superb collection of minds focused on the cause of my present difficulty.

Currently, I am under the care of Dr. Mark Gilbert, the NCI doctor who was actually leading the conference, mobilizing the effort to find a cure for oligodendrogliomas and other types of rare brain tumors.

Dr. Berger joined us and the Dabbieres for a video call during a break in the rare tumor conference and gave his opinion that surgery was definitely appropriate in my case.

"It's important to clear out all of the enhanced area of the tumor," he said. "Including resecting as much of the remaining tumor as possible."

Of course, Kim and I cast our net wide, seeking additional opinions. Ultimately, my doctors at NIH also saw surgery as the proper course of action and knew of Dr. Berger as one of the top brain surgeons in the world. We felt greater comfort because Hopkins also ultimately agreed that surgery would be a reasonable thing to do under the circumstances, with radiation and chemotherapy to follow.

Analysis of the tumor post-surgery would ultimately determine whether radiation and chemo were necessary. We heard once again that doctors, until they actually access the specific area of the brain, can only speculate about the grade and genetic makeup of a tumor. In this day and age, again, it seems a little crude to have to resort to opening one's head to figure out a tumor's true nature, but that apparently remains the case.

We decided to go forward with Dr. Berger. He was ably supported by his UCSF colleagues, Dr. Susan Chang, the head of Neuro-Oncology, and Dr. Javier Villanueva-Meyer, the head of Neuroradiology. Given the bleed that occurred during my first surgery, Dr. Berger recommended further blood testing. I appreciated that recommendation, as I had been thinking about what had caused the bleed after my first surgery.

Amid the flurry of preparations for going into my second surgery, as directed by Dr. Berger, I went to see the hematologist again who ran a battery of blood tests. In December 2018, the hematologist revealed the likely reason for the post-surgical disaster I suffered in 2015 after my first brain surgery. He said that I had a mild form of hemophilia, a lack of certain clotting factor that caused the bleeding that almost killed me.

I possessed only the most general idea of what hemophilia was all about. If I thought about it at all, I assumed it was a tragic condition affecting people where if they prick their finger and bleed, they would run into serious bleeding problems. I knew hemophilia ran in the bloodlines of the Romanovs, the doomed Russian royal family.

But looking back, the diagnosis made sense. As a kid I always bruised easily, and the bruises seemed to linger longer when compared to other people. I didn't think all that much about it.

I played sports and led a very energetic childhood. Bumps and bruises just came with the territory.

But the undiagnosed condition remained with me as I grew up. It turns out that the blood running through my veins was lacking in certain clotting factors. I had lived my whole life up until that point without knowing anything about it.

Thinking back about my entire situation from the start struck me as extraordinary. I had walked into Hopkins on the morning of the surgery, no wheelchair, no obvious impairment. I actually thought I looked pretty good. I had always tried to stay fit, and led a fairly active lifestyle—skiing, running, biking, and golfing. Five years prior to my surgery, when I had turned fifty, I competed in a seventy-five mile bike race in New York City and New Jersey without a problem.

But I rode in ignorance. At the time of the race, I apparently already had a sizable tumor in my brain, as well as a blood condition that would make brain surgery a serious problem.

It's a frightening proposition, the idea that we can go about our days and ways without knowing that we have the specific seeds of mortality within us. In my professional life, I spent three decades traveling frequently to the Middle East and South America, flying to time zones seven or eight hours removed from home, in a profession that requires a lot of energy, thinking, and long hours. I wasn't exactly Superman, Spartacus, or Ironman. But I was a reasonably fit adult male, and I always tolerated time zone changes well.

Perhaps being in pretty good shape and having the mindset I developed from wrestling helped save my life. I'll never really know, but the background couldn't have hurt. I do know this: I had walked into the hospital on my own two feet and left in an ambulance.

There I was five years later facing a second brain surgery at UCSF with Dr. Berger operating. I was comforted by the fact that Dr. Berger was well aware of my hemophilia results and was prepared for the problem.

I wrote to Dr. Berger a week or so before my second surgery was scheduled. I wanted to make sure he knew that I was a "glass half full" kind of guy, and he responded that he was the same way. I informed him that I totally appreciated the risks involved in the type of surgery he'd be undertaking. I felt like hearing repeated warnings about surgical risks was bad karma.

I had already signed a lot of consent forms, acknowledging that I was at risk of not surviving the operation. Having been a lawyer for a long time, I knew that a place like UCSF most likely has very good legal representation. The consent forms were not optional. At the same time, I knew choosing not to have surgery was really not an option, either. But when it comes down to it, it's really not all too difficult to craft a consent form which explains that you might die from the surgery.

Even so, my family and I were still hearing about the risks of surgery right up until the moment I was being wheeled into the operating room. I preferred that my children not be exposed to the warnings but they were. I felt badly because I really had no opportunity to explain to my children that they shouldn't worry because my blood-clotting issues would be addressed, so the second surgery would be more straightforward than the first.

I didn't feel especially worried. I had total confidence in Dr. Berger.

As it turned out, my second craniotomy, at UCSF on January 3, 2019, could not have gone more smoothly. I felt the odds were in my favor to have a flawless surgery. Before my surgery, the chief of hematology at UCSF gave me a blood clotting treatment. Dr. Berger then performed the second craniotomy over a six-hour period. There was no abnormal bleeding that time around, no additional blood infusions were needed, and Dr. Berger was able to resect the entire enhanced area, including most of my tumor.

Seemingly moments later, I recall surfacing from the surgery to see my family surrounding me. Indeed the operation had occurred. I felt pretty good, considering—a little nauseous, maybe, but no real headache. I was pretty certain that the anesthesia, the meds, and the IVs caused what little discomfort I had, while also preventing most of the pain.

Later that afternoon following the surgery, Dr. Berger explained that during the procedure he felt it vital to resect the enhanced five-millimeter area and "clear out" the residual tumor.

Miraculously, I was discharged from UCSF just two days after my admission. The difference between my first surgery and my second was like night and day. To go from a two month stay in two hospitals and lots of rehabilitation to a two-day stay in a single hospital and no rehab, represented one of the happiest developments of my life. It's hard to describe the emotions associated with my rehabilitation, which remained painfully fresh in my mind.

But we didn't want to take any chances. Hoping for the best, but preparing for the worst, we made a decision that made us feel much more comfortable about my post-surgical recovery.

Chapter Nine

Surgery with No Complications, and the Beauty of the Pacific Coast!

I was free. Whatever was happening inside my brain, regardless of whether the second operation had rooted out almost all of the tumor and had removed the lit-up section, I stood on my own two feet the evening of the surgery. I still couldn't believe I had been released from the hospital so quickly, but I was glad to be up and out of the hospital.

We decided there was no way we were budging from San Francisco. I wanted to stay close to UCSF, just in case something went wrong. The doctors had also instructed me not to fly for five days following my surgery, so I was pretty much marooned anyway.

Kim, the kids, and I stayed at an Airbnb very close to the hospital. Thankfully, I received clearance from Dr. Berger's professional staff to exercise. I always loved walking the hills in San Francisco, and began doing short circuits starting three days after my surgery. It tired me out a bit, but I still appreciated the fact that I could actually venture outside.

San Francisco, of course, is one of the best places in the country for walking hills. At the corresponding point in the aftermath of my first surgery, I was sunk deep in a coma. Even after I was finally back on my feet, walking was my therapy of choice.

I enjoyed the visits and company of a couple of friends and clients, happily breaking bread with them. Despite the great joy I felt from guests dropping by, I never lost sight of the need to stay close to my doctors at UCSF in the event a problem arose.

I did some follow-up blood testing at UCSF and the results all came back clean. A week to the day after my second surgery, I was ready to move on to the final recovery stage. I felt as if relocating to some place very special was in order.

Given everything we'd been through, beginning in December 2014, my first touch-and-go hospital stay, my near-death experience, extensive rehabilitation at NRH, the finding of hemophilia, and now the second craniotomy in 2019 on the West Coast, we thought we deserved to spend some quality time at a nice recuperation spot.

The coastal town of Half Moon Bay nestles in the low cliffs above the Pacific, about forty-five minutes south of San Francisco. The town is well-known for the challenging Mavericks surfing area, nearby in rough seas off Pilar Point Harbor. The spectacular winter surfing attracts big wave daredevils and is definitely not for the faint of heart, with surf that routinely crests at fifty feet or more. When the towering waves break, the crash can be picked up on earthquake sensors.

For me, Kim, Garrett, and Taylor, the scenery had a bracing grandeur that seemed to call me back to life. I was alive, and I told myself that these were the kinds of things I lived for—my family, great natural beauty, and recovering my health. The views of the ocean from our hotel at Half Moon Bay were extraordinary. The surf toppled and tumbled off shore. Majestic to look at, but not anything I felt like challenging. Fresh off a second brain surgery, I felt I had endured enough challenges to last a lifetime.

Another local feature lured me more successfully. Our amazing walks on the beach brought us past Half Moon Bay Golf Links. I enjoy playing golf, but I was under doctor's orders not to indulge. Given the beauty of the course and the stunning natural backdrop, it was torture to totally skip the sport. "A good walk ruined" is the golfer's rueful description of the game—and there I was, limited simply to the good walk, unspoiled by shanks, slices, and hooks.

I didn't see myself as violating doctor's orders if I allowed myself a couple of chip shots to the green. Approaching the club pro, I mentioned my recent brain surgery and told him it would be great if I could take a couple swings as something of a gift for all I had been through.

"Maybe just a short shot pitching a wedge up to the eighteenth green?" I suggested. The pro happily obliged.

The experience felt invigorating, a truly amazing step in my recovery. I realized one's bucket list changes depending on the circumstances one has been through. The fact that our stay at Half Moon Bay followed just six days after my second craniotomy supercharged my mood. There was no way I wasn't going to take a few chip shots to celebrate the victory over the greatest health challenge of my life.

We had some great meals, great walks, and great sleep. We finished up our trip on January 14, 2019 and flew back to Maryland late that afternoon. We made it back home in one piece. Everything seemed like a miracle: the beauty of the

Pacific, golf, air travel, as well as the fact that in our absence our house had remained in one piece. It seems we had dodged a big East Coast snow storm. We took that bonus, too! In fact, after surviving brain surgery everything seemed like a bonus.

"Nothing is so sweet as to return from the sea," says the Greek poet Homer, "and to listen to the rain on the rooftop of home." I had not actually been out to sea, of course, but I felt as though I was returning from quite a voyage. I was coming back home, coming back to myself, coming back to life.

On the first Sunday after our return—January 20, 2019—we hosted a brunch at our home. We wanted to express our appreciation to our family and friends who had been so supportive over the course of the entire crisis. Words can't explain how grateful we were for all of the encouragement we received. We hadn't yet seen anyone since before we left for San Francisco. The get-together gave us the opportunity to give big hugs to a lot of family and friends, and we couldn't have been more pleased to express our heartfelt appreciation to so many great and caring people.

Again, as with lofting the ball onto the eighteenth green of Half Moon Bay Golf Links, everything old seemed new again. My home, family, and old friends—it was all hard to beat. The phrase "new lease on life" occurred to me during that brunch. Somehow, the fact that I still had to do a course of radiation and chemotherapy didn't dampen Kim's and my shared enthusiasm for hosting our family and friends.

All through that extraordinary day, I experienced the gratitude of a survivor, incredibly thankful to be alive following a second brain surgery, to dodge a second bullet, and to avoid the potential adverse implications of surgery. To be with so many great family members and friends felt like a tremendous gift of love. I resolved to be there for my family, of course, but also for our friends, should they ever end up in a crisis of any sort. It takes a village, as they say.

*   *   *

To make a sports analogy, I felt like I had come from behind and pulled off a big victory in the final game of a major tournament. I suppose comparing my situation to a sporting event is hardly doing justice to my speedy recovery. However, my son and I have always used a "last thirty seconds of a match" come-from-behind analogy whenever we needed to achieve a difficult task.

Chapter Ten

Next Steps—Radiation, Chemotherapy, and Alternative Therapies

The good feelings from that get-together at our home gave me further strength and motivation to tackle my next challenge, which was understanding and choosing among the options for radiation and chemotherapy. The hope for the regimen (at least in my mind) would be to shrink what remained of the tumor, thus freeing me of my haunting problem.

Kim and I consulted with Dr. Mark Gilbert, whom we had previously heard from during the November conference on oligo-dendrogliomas. Dr. Gilbert is the chief of the Neuro-Oncology Branch at National Cancer Institute (NCI), which is part of the National Institutes of Health (NIH).

Radiation

The radiation part of the post-operative treatment was, of course, brand new to me. I had to be sized for a protective mask that I would wear during the procedure. The purpose of the mask was to make sure my head stayed properly positioned to receive the radiation. It was a fairly short outpatient procedure, but I had to do it five days a week for six weeks straight. I made my way every week to NIH to visit with my new friends in the radiation department.

For the treatment, I would lie down and the nurse or technician would put my protective mask in place and get me properly positioned to receive the radiation. Once the procedure began, I would typically fall asleep as I stretched out for the therapy.

I was prepared for my hair to fall out. As expected, it fell out around the radiation site. To avoid the appearance of an alien crop circle on my scalp, I decided to head off the inevitable by shaving my head.

Radiation treatment for these tumors can be either more focused (proton beams) or less focused (photon beams) depending on the opinion of the oncologist. Dr. Gilbert recommended a less focused beam, since the tumor diffused itself, and the aim was to radiate as much of the affected tissue as possible.

Every patient is different, and treatment recommendations vary. For example, Brock Greene, one of the major fundraisers for oligodendroglioma research (he's the founder of OligoNation), has two sons that have the same tumor I have, but their treatment employed a more focused beam.

The proton beam was recommended for the Greens by top doctors at Sloan Kettering. Adding a bit more uncertainty to our thinking, the physician team at NIH proposed that I undergo treatment with the less focused Photon beam. These are the kind of almost unanswerable dilemmas that often cropped up throughout my medical crisis.

One side effect from the month-and-a-half long course of radiation was that my speech capabilities seemed to be decaying. I found it difficult to speak without slurring. So the doctors prescribed a course of the steroid Prednisone to reduce the inflammation. That seemed to have some benefit.

NIH was just a few miles from my house. As I really found walking more and more enjoyable and cathartic, I walked back home from NIH a number of times after the radiation therapy. It was winter and still cold, but I felt as if I needed to unwind a bit after the treatment, so I really enjoyed the walk.

By the end of this six-week process, I had become quite friendly with the nurses, technician, and the lead radiation doctor managing my treatment. The NIH group presented me with a certificate for being a proud radiation treatment graduate. I took several photographs with my NIH radiation team. The treatment was very important to me—the certificate, not so important. What I really wanted was for the cancer to vanish from my brain.

We've all heard the horror stories about chemotherapy, the next step in my treatment. Tales of nausea, disorientation, exhaustion, and other side effects abound. I felt as though I were a marathon runner hitting "the wall" at the twentieth mile. But I accepted the necessity of chemo.

I did wonder about other, less extreme approaches, such as those offered in the realm of alternative medicine. The pharmaceutical folks and the medical world seemed less enthusiastic about those, as there were few medical studies on the value of holistic treatments. I had always heard the suggestion that holistic medicine has not been heavily researched. One problem is that no one can take out a patent on bee venom, mushrooms, broccoli, or other natural remedies. Of course, no patent means that there is no clear way to monetize a treatment. Pardon my somewhat jaundiced views of what is available medically to address cancer.

Radiation and chemo have generally been the accepted standard of care for the past twenty or so years. I dutifully proceeded with the prescribed regimens. Some research did indeed correlate the success of chemo with the genetic makeup of my tumor.

Despite my frustration with the lack of support for alternative therapies, I was getting a better understanding of why traditional and alternative approaches didn't coordinate, but rather were often at odds with one another. Maybe I'm less of a believer in Eastern medicines because, for example, they didn't seem to work for me. In the years between my two surgeries, I experimented with one of these therapies: acupuncture.

But perhaps the energy flow theories of Eastern medicine applied to my case without me even realizing it. Does alternative medicine work or not? As far as I'm concerned, the jury is still out. All I know is that acupuncture was expensive, not covered by my health insurance, and did not prevent me from having a second brain surgery.

I will say, though, that I do eat a lot of the veggies that the holistic world suggests are helpful, like broccoli, mushrooms, garlic, and lentils. In short, I generally eat a whole food, plant-based diet. I try to minimize red meats and eat a fair amount of fish. I guess diet is one of the areas where I feel like I do have some control. And certainly, I just feel better eating a healthier diet.

Chemotherapy
As far as the specific chemotherapy treatment, we really didn't understand which option might be the better choice. The

decision came down to two main methods—Temodar or PCV. Our research indicated that PCV had terrible side effects and that people have trouble tolerating the full set of treatment rounds. Kim and I discussed the two treatment options with Dr. Susan Chang, director of Neuro-Oncology at UCSF. Although we were initially heading in the direction of Temodar, we ultimately decided to go with PCV. A big deciding factor was the recommendation of PCV by Dr. Gilbert of NIH. He indicated that there were several studies that supported the use of PCV in connection with treating my particular type of tumor.

The three drugs involved are Procarbazine, Lomustine, and Vincristine. Under the direction of Dr. Gilbert, the NIH modified the regimen by omitting Vincristine—so my chemo was actually PC, rather than PCV. Apparently the "V" part of the formulation had a lot of troublesome side effects, and there was no evidence that Vincristine added real value.

The end result was that I found myself starting on the exact type of treatment—chemotherapy—that I had been attempting to avoid for the last several years. I haven't heard much enthusiasm from former patients about chemo. To the contrary, there seems to be endless amounts of information online, suggesting that radiation and chemotherapy are pushed by the deep-pocketed pharmaceutical companies that have put all their research money into chemotherapy as the most effective course of treatment.

I wasn't ready to buy into such dark conspiracy theories about "Big Pharma," and could not have summoned the energy to investigate them anyway. The bottom line was that we just decided to move forward with chemotherapy as the current standard of care.

The specialists to whom I entrusted my post-operative care were an incredible team: Dr. Gilbert (NIH), Dr. Chang (UCSF), and Dr. Laterra (Hopkins). I wasn't going to doubt their advice. The team recommended that radiation and chemotherapy were the ways to go, based on their effectiveness for the specific genetic composition of my tumor. I was glad to hear that the frequently slow march of medicine had reached such an advanced point that the molecular composition of a tumor could predict the odds of success for suggested treatments. Peering into cell structures and DNA at the atomic level was really getting down to the nitty gritty!

Under the direct guidance of Dr. Gilbert and Dr. Byram Ozer of Hopkins/Sibley, I underwent a full course of chemo. Dr. Ozer is my Neuro-Oncologist at Sibley, where the chemo was administered. I will say this: Securing the medications and dealing with insurance issues, following the prescribed schedule, and taking the proper medications almost wore me out. I'm fairly certain that the effects of the medication, and not the process of securing the medication, are what are supposed to wear you down. Ultimately I went through a four-month long chemotherapy regimen. Chemotherapy medication is considered a hazardous waste for non-patients and can cause skin irritation and other conditions. So I had to be particularly careful not to contaminate and infect my family during the whole process.

I consider myself lucky in that none of the extreme side effects I had read or heard about seemed to come true in my case. Chemo tired me out a bit. I felt a little faded, as if the phrase "a shadow of my former self" was coming true. The chemo also may have affected my memory.

But I survived. (As I write these words, I'm looking around for a piece of wood on which to knock.)

Throughout my life, I've always had my own views on the significance of philosophy and religion as they relate to medical care. Maybe all of the medical trials and tribulations I endured had suddenly made a believer out of me? That seemed opportunistic and weak. I didn't like to think that I was proof of the old adage, "there are no atheists in the foxhole." But I have indeed headed in that direction, yet with some measure of my "lawyer's logic" applied to the situation. I will say this: Our family never used to say prayers before meals. After all we've been through, you can bet we now say prayers for good health and happiness before every meal.

Do I now subscribe to the miraculous? I am definitely more willing to see small marvels and wondrous circumstances wherever I go. (Even a car accident leading to a life-saving cancer diagnosis? What are the odds of that?) In the proper frame of mind, every sunrise is a miracle. But some supposedly random occurrences seem to hold greater significance for me than they used to.

For example, Dr. Gilbert's office is located in Building 37 on the sprawling NIH campus. It did not escape me that I knew Building 37 intimately before I had ever become Dr. Gilbert's patient or had ever heard his name. My familiarity had nothing to do with medicine, doctors, or brain cancer. Early on in my legal career, when Building 37 was being built, I negotiated the design and construction contracts for it. It happens to sit in a prominent location on the NIH campus—at the main entrance to NIH. In my case, what goes around came around in a quite unexpected way.

I also hope I'll be able to say that my brain tumor was cured in the same building that I helped usher into existence as a lawyer, some twenty years ago. Don't even think of telling me that my conclusion is neither reasonable nor logical. I won't put a smiley face here because I've never seen one in a published book. Let's just wait for another miracle to occur!

PART TWO

From Darkness to Enlightenment

Chapter Eleven
Achieving a Better Perspective

Many times, the truth becomes clear only in the aftermath. I've been fortunate to have had some successes in life, but the achievements that are most vivid in my mind arose quite quickly out of my medical crisis. Among them were my recognition as the sickest person on the neuro intensive care unit and my insurer's characterization of me as a "catastrophic loss." The attorney assisting me in social security disability matters said that he had never seen the Social Security Administration approve a disability claim so quickly. Frankly, I found the speedy approval of my disability claim to be a bit frightening.

These are the kind of achievements that I'd just as soon not receive. Except for being afflicted with a brain tumor—and that's a pretty big "except"—I've been fortunate in the way life has played out. My thoughts always tend toward the positive. I appreciate the analogy here to the old line about Mary Todd Lincoln: "Other than that, Mrs. Lincoln, how did you like the play?"

But my recent experience, as awful as it has been, has given me the great gift of perspective. The aftermath has included the process of adapting to a "new me." It has allowed me to reflect on how I approached my education, my career, and my life in general. It's also given me the time to consider how my past may have shaped the way I approached academics and relationships with my friends, colleagues, and family. Above all, I've had a chance to think more carefully about the ins and outs of the vital task of parenting.

The catalog of what I went through to put me where I am today is pretty daunting. I survived two brain surgeries, a coma, life support, life-threatening complications, years of rehabilitative therapy, a diagnosis of hemophilia, seemingly endless MRIs, and regimens of radiation and chemotherapy. I had to relearn how to walk, speak, and think. Each one of these trials were, plain and simple, life-altering events.

I now feel like a greater power has granted me both the time and the hard-won experience to write this account. As they say, I've been through hell and back. Now I feel obligated to write about my experience in the hope that I might actually help people.

Many others have undergone similar trials, and a few have detailed what happened to them. I wish I could say that I underwent some extraordinary metaphysical event, where I visited heaven, for example, or saw myself floating above my own body while lying comatose in bed. That didn't happen for me—or at least, I don't recall it. I was laid out in the hospital, unresponsive, with nothing much going on mentally. That might make for a less grandiose story, but at the same time I have to think that the life lessons I've learned have been eminently worthwhile.

While I lacked noteworthy out-of-body experiences, I do recall a friend stopping by our home several months after my first surgery as I was still recuperating.

"I think we may have our old Bob Brams back," she said as she left our home. She said that to Kim, not to me.

When my wife relayed the comment to me, I was of two minds. On the one hand, I was glad to hear that I was perceived as being back in the picture. But I was also a little troubled to learn that I had been perceived as "not all there" for months. It represented a curt reminder of what should have already been extremely obvious to me: I had been essentially off the planet for quite a while.

Recently I ran across an anonymous post on the internet, which addresses a salient truth about recovery from brain surgery:

> I think the hardest part of cancer treatment is what seems to be the end. Everyone assumes you're 'cured' and you no longer need their help. However, like a soldier at the end of a war, you still do need help putting your life back together, complicated by the fact that you're not cured.

I live with a cavity in my brain the size of an infant's fist. While I'm now dealing with various physical impediments and trying to adapt to them, I do feel as though I essentially have the same personality as I did when I had my full brain. I'd like to think that my personality is, in fact, more stable with much of the tumor gone and without the pressure and stress of the practice of law.

My family might debate me on the issue of whether my old personality is back. But my life's circumstances have now changed in many significant ways. I'm no longer faced with endless work pressures, a busy schedule, and client demands, as well as regular international travel. In my more than thirty years of practice, I don't think a day went by, including during vacations, where I didn't check my work emails regularly. I was going through a lot of juggling and pressure. For example: working on a motion that was required to be filed on January 2 while on a cruise ship. Unfortunate, but the deadline had to be met. I'm now trying to lead a much more stress-free lifestyle. I try to keep to a minimum all demands on my time, which formerly were nearly constant. I'll probably never know what caused my tumor, but I doubt living with a high degree of stress helped.

During my professional career, I never really felt that work pressures bothered me physically or mentally. In fact, I seemed to thrive on a busy schedule. Maybe it gave me a sense of purpose. Now I'm not sure the hectic life I formerly led was healthy at all. The normal wide array of ordinary, everyday stresses and strains can appear a little crazy, as soon as you step away from them and gain perspective. I've always heard the modern routine characterized as "being nibbled to death by ducks."

Currently I've involuntarily taken on a very different type of pressure—surviving my health crisis. It's more focused and single-minded. So far, I've been pretty good at dealing with this pressure and uncertainty. I haven't allowed it to overwhelm me. That said, thoughts about my health always seem to linger in my mind.

When I boil it down, and given what I've been through and still go through, I realize my life can never be the same as it was before my surgery. I can't help but harbor a hope that my tumor will somehow shrink and go away and I'll be free of this haunting problem. While I stay optimistic, I don't see the tumor magically vanishing.

While my health situation stays on my mind, I make it a point not to get discouraged. Sure, I suffer from the after-effects of a cancer diagnosis. I feel dizzy from time to time, and tire very easily. I try to let the situation motivate me and give me greater strength to try to achieve more valuable goals and—since the clock is ticking—achieve them more quickly. Summoning this strength seems to help me minimize the consequences of various post-operative repercussions. I'm well aware that the clock is, of course, ticking for all of us. Sadly, the alarm has sounded for over three million people (as of the time of writing) that have passed away due to the COVID-19 pandemic.

Brain cancer changed me in a lot of ways, some of them quite annoying. But what I want to concentrate on here, and what I want to communicate in the remainder of this book, is the new perspective it has given me. With the clutter of day-to-day responsibilities cleared away, what remains is precious. I feel that I can assess experiences that were once obscured by the hum-drum everyday rush and see their value (or the lack thereof) much more clearly. One thing that has become particularly clear is my need to nap and hold off on speaking before I go out or try to do anything. Without the rest, I find it more difficult to speak and function effectively. And it has become quite clear to me, unfortunately, that speaking and projecting my voice tire me out very quickly.

My health setback and subsequent disability have caused me to think more about my need, indeed my obligation, to serve a greater purpose. It's a motivation that I didn't really have while making a living as a lawyer. In short, my experience has sharpened my focus on helping others and fostering a greater sense of community.

The life lessons I've brought forward are not limited to those gleaned from my medical crisis. I now see my new career (helping in the fight against cancer) in a clearer light. I understand human aspects of the law in ways I never have before. I want to accomplish things in the world that serve a far greater purpose than the narrow scope of what I focused on as a lawyer.

What did I learn over three decades of dealing with clients, determining the legal ramifications of large-scale construction projects, and negotiating the minutiae of complex contracts? What I was focused on as a lawyer in the past was of the utmost importance to my clients and to me at the time. But some of those lessons from law carry forward and apply to my new focus on service and helping others. I was effective as a lawyer. But, I now want to harness my old skills to face the fresh challenges of helping to support the fight against cancer. The cancer fight confronts me and countless others every day.

My health experience has also impacted the way I think as a parent. I've come to recognize goals that are far more important than providing material items to my children. My perspective has become clearer. I feel the urge to give guidance to my children on complex events or situations that I better appreciate and understand.

Sometimes you have to give your children some perspective—that what they are worrying about is really not that important in the overall scheme of things. But it's helpful to be able to give these issues some greater thought. No one in the world has the interest of our children more at heart than we do as parents.

I also find the uncertainty I face to be unusual and quite a bit different from the uncertainty and risks we all confront all the time. The situation prompts me to think about and pursue my goals with some haste. It always struck me how much more clearly and effectively we all think (or at least, I think) as a deadline gets closer. For me, a clear and present deadline influences every day and every thought. I'm hoping the urgency that I now feel will better refine my thoughts and that they now have more value for readers. The bottom line is that things are not perfect for me, but the alternative would have been far worse.

Chapter Twelve

There's More than One Path from Average to Excellence

I grew up in a warm and loving household, first in Wilmington, Delaware, and then in Chadds Ford, Pennsylvania. I had wonderful and caring parents and a great older brother, Jon. My father was a physician and my mother was my father's office manager. My brother is a technical writer for a software company. My father was a Rutgers and Jefferson Medical School graduate, and both my mother and brother graduated from the University of Pennsylvania. I have none of the usual complaints about a troubled childhood and was a happy and well-adjusted kid. However, I still managed to make things more difficult for myself in school.

I was fortunate to have a number of good friends and stayed busy doing a variety of activities. But I was not as focused as I should have been on the academic front. In elementary and middle school my grades were always about average. I suspect my teachers might have rated my academic performance as "meh."

There seemed a strange inevitability to my classroom work in elementary and middle school. I'd rise from my desk after a test believing I had done fairly well. I should have realized that my cheery optimism was almost a sure sign that I had actually done poorly. When I got my test paper back, I'd see that, sure enough, I had turned in an average performance.

My grades weren't a case of a "gentleman's C," as George W. Bush described it. Mine were an underachiever's C. My grades improved in high school. However, I stumbled back to the C range at the start of college. While, of course, I didn't like receiving poor grades, I don't recall it discouraging me from trying to do better the next time. With hindsight I realize that my focus was still a bit off.

Later on, in college, I began to figure out that I needed to concentrate harder on what I was going to be tested on, rather than on what I understood easily or what I enjoyed most. I also needed to learn to dig deeper on subjects and to develop the patience to fully work through problems.

Growing up, sports seemed far more important to me than academics. But even in the athletic arena, although I came around to being pretty good at sports as a kid, I frequently started out poorly and had a number of uninspired seasons. One year, playing Little League baseball, I struck out almost every time I came to the plate. As a ninth grader, I lost every wrestling match. Actually, to be strictly accurate, I tied one match and lost all the others. With all the losses, the tie felt like a victory.

My performances should have been kind of embarrassing, but I don't recall feeling that way. The failures never prevented me from sticking with the sport. It never really entered my mind to quit or do something other than just try to improve at the sports I had chosen.

The takeaway from this is that children are pretty resilient. Parents don't need to whisk their children into another activity when they don't do well early on and seem frustrated or unhappy. While it doesn't always make sense intuitively, we seem to learn best by failing and experiencing frustration and overcoming the failure.

In fact, numerous surveys have determined why children like to participate in athletics. Surprisingly, kids rarely list "winning" as their top reason. Rather, "getting better at my sport" is almost always the number one motivator. This seems to hold true across all fields of endeavor and for people of all ages. Quite simply, improving at any activity represents a favorite aspect of life for most human beings.

Adults should avoid imposing their own judgments and feelings on their children. Our children may have a better balance of determination and blissful ignorance than we adults might think. As parents, maybe it's best to fight the temptation to be overly protective. Doing things for our children that they are capable of doing themselves does nothing to help them to grow up and become independent. Just like adults, kids probably feel better about themselves and gain confidence after they've figured out a solution to their own problems.

Despite (or perhaps because of) some early struggles, I improved. I ended up as a starter on my high school's varsity soccer, wrestling, and baseball teams, and was made captain of the wrestling team. Though I had an inauspicious start, I turned out to be one of the school's best wrestlers.

While Delaware is a small state, it does have a pool of fairly solid wrestling talent. I was thrilled to win my qualifying tournament for the state tournament. In fact, I was the only wrestler on the team who qualified, and I wound up ranked as one of the top eight wrestlers in the state in my weight class. I was honored as a senior to be named the team's Outstanding Wrestler, and my high school's Outstanding Senior Athlete.

Now, almost forty years later, I understand that a plaque still hangs at the school with my senior athlete award. For what it's worth, I've got that going for me.

Reflecting on that period, I can readily believe that, after experiencing so much frustration and failure, my ultimate success in sports gave me a tremendous boost of confidence in many areas. I carried a sense of achievement with me later on, and it ended up helping me with activities having nothing to do with sports.

Participating and competing in sports seemed much more important to me in high school than academics—maybe an attitude that was short-sighted. But maybe not. I played three sports for four years, enjoyed myself, and ended up as a B student in high school. I do think participation in sports for so long made me a more competitive person. I knew what winning felt like. At the very least, I was well-rounded, though I never recall seeing academics as a competitive activity. For example, I didn't think of myself as someone who needed to finish at the top of my class. I never really felt like that was my place, and it really didn't seem that important to me.

For reasons that still escape me, my high school didn't have final exams when I was a student there. Although I wasn't walking the halls at the time clamoring for finals, it might have been helpful to develop the ability to study and more thoroughly understand a full semester's worth of material. As a result, I didn't feel particularly well-prepared for the academic rigors of college, and certainly not for finals. (My high school now has finals.)

After high school, I attended Muhlenberg College, a small liberal arts school in Allentown, Pennsylvania. I still had not quite figured out how to study or persevere in academics as effectively as I needed to succeed at that next level. I joined a fraternity and stayed active in sports, starting on the wrestling team for two years at Muhlenberg. While I definitely don't have the lean build of a top runner, I also ran cross-country in my junior year to get in shape for wrestling.

I was a business major, but I had no real path in mind for life or work. In my freshman year of college my grades were at a C/C+ level. Ultimately, I cracked a B average for grades by graduation, but not without making a concerted effort to pull off a number of As in my senior year. As in high school, I never felt particularly inspired by academics. Perhaps I just never thought I was smart enough to get top grades. A "B" was good enough.

As I approached the end of college, I didn't feel quite ready to jump into the real world. For no good reason other than I thought I could make fairly logical, reasonable, and compelling arguments, law school seemed like it might be an interesting challenge. I ended up at the University of Bridgeport School of Law.

I once again found myself in a fairly recognizable place academically—somewhere in the middle of the pack, rather than near the top. And yet looking back, I can't recall ever thinking that I couldn't succeed in law school. To the contrary, I graduated from college feeling confident that I could do well in law school, the legal profession, and in life. I saw law school as a new start. Perhaps it was a benefit of my optimism, coupled with blissful ignorance of the challenges I would face in the study and practice of law.

Today, kids customarily visit their schools once or twice before committing to attend. That wasn't my path. I didn't see my first law school until a day or so before classes started. I'm not sure why I had that attitude, but I never felt a pressing need to visit a school before going there. I didn't see law school as occupying all that much time, and I really looked at it as simply a means to an end—maybe not the best way to look at it.

My idiosyncratic approach to legal education continued as I cycled through not one, not two, but three law schools. While I graduated from the University of Bridgeport Law School, I attended both Georgetown University Law Center and Catholic University Law School as a visiting student. At the same time I was going to school in DC, I also worked in legal settings. I found that I really enjoyed the combination of work and law school. I suppose it all created a structure for me that was almost calming in a way.

This was far from the standard path to a sterling career in law. But it worked for me, and beyond that, it taught me that the standard path is not always the best for everyone. Human beings are not cookies, and the cookie cutter method isn't universally successful.

Although I'm not sure I could have articulated my belief at the time, I had an intuitive sense that making strong connections with people was an important aspect of my education. I've always tended to value relationships over a focus on academics. My earlier experience in sports helped me to form good friendships during the course of my middle, high school, and college years. Indeed, I developed several friendships from my earliest days in middle school that I still value very much today. In fact, an old friend going back to sixth grade stopped by to visit me after my second surgery in San Francisco.

I had worked hard to improve my grades in my last year of college, but I learned that law schools didn't give much consideration to senior year grades. For admission decisions, law schools certainly didn't care if you had good common sense. Interestingly, I consider common sense to be one of the more valuable assets I had to offer in the practice of law.

I'm not quite sure why, but again, I didn't really prepare well for the LSAT. As a result, I had neither the best grades nor stellar LSAT results. I've come to believe that my average academic performance and my mindset generally caused me to want to focus on "real world" problems as opposed to solving the "academic hypotheticals" at the end of each of the chapters of many of my law school texts.

Students who excel in high school readily accept grades as the primary marker of their success. But I found the ground shifts a bit in graduate school as one begins thinking about entering the working world. One important element of success in higher education and beyond is having the ability to build relationships, especially good mentor relationships. Such personal bonds become valuable to gain real life experience and for securing letters of recommendation. But they will also forge the interpersonal skills that are necessary to succeed in all manner of endeavors. I found real value in being able to get along well with people in both work and social settings.

A prime example of this is a relationship I developed during law school while serving as an intern for a federal judge. This represented my first taste of real-world, hands-on experience. It demonstrated that I could show up, engage with others on a professional level, and be effective in a work environment. I felt like these achievements were much more important to my development than just sitting through law school classes. In that work environment, it felt very important to me to do "A" caliber work. But it also was helpful that the judge and I got along well and had similar values.

Perhaps I'm rationalizing my average academic performance, but I think I was just getting a little bit tired of the routine of school work, and it didn't seem incredibly meaningful or valuable to me once I understood the basic principles of law. I just wanted to finish law school, take the bar exam, and get on with the real work of helping clients address their problems. I'm not suggesting that one shouldn't worry about performing well academically from the start of high school and throughout college. Of course students should always strive to perform their best and persevere in school. For any meaningful job, employers will review college and graduate school grades and coursework when making hiring decisions. When sifting through resumes, potential employers may just toss yours aside if your GPA is too low, or if you didn't go to a top law school or if you didn't make law review.

However, if things don't play out well academically, don't assume that all is lost. Instead, one may have to work harder to develop better contacts with potential employers, build strengths and skills that potential employers see as valuable, and always strive to do superior work. As mentioned, I never overlooked the importance of applying good common sense in all of my cases. I have always told my children, in real life you have to get an "A" on *all* your work.

Chapter Thirteen

Finding Your Passion by Respecting Your Interests and Successes

When you pass the bar exam, you're qualified to practice law. If you fail, you're stuck taking the exam again—and again. The prime example of this situation is the late John F. Kennedy Jr., who failed twice and passed the exam only on his third attempt. A lot of people have struck out on their first tries—Franklin Roosevelt, Hillary Clinton, and Michelle Obama, to name only three notables. The nationwide failure rate hovers around 25 percent.

Passing the bar on my first try helped reaffirm the idea that I have the aptitude for the legal profession. Pretty early on during my rigorous study for the exam, it became a "no brainer" (of course, pun intended) for me to conclude that I never, ever wanted to put in the study time again for the bar exam. Of all the tests I've encountered in my life, I viewed that one as a competitive effort with very real consequences. Failing the bar was simply not an option. Even though I'm sure that I would have kept taking the bar exam until I passed, I'm also of the view that failing the exam may have caused me to doubt my legal skills.

After passing the bar and becoming an attorney, I was fortunate enough to land a clerkship with the same federal judge for whom I had interned, apparently having successfully proven my legal skills as an intern. The judge was candid, saying that had I not passed the bar, she would not have hired me as a clerk. It was a little sobering to hear that, but I understood. The judge's view was that I might be distracted from my clerkship work by further studies for a second try at the exam.

While clerking, I found myself surrounded by attorneys who had graduated at the top of their classes from the best law schools in the country. I did wonder if I could cut it in my new clerking job, but I knew that I had already performed well as an intern. I never recall doubting my intelligence, my ability to write clearly, or my ability to work hard whenever I needed to find the right solution to a problem.

Over the years, several colleagues from my clerkship have become good friends. One of my closest friends is a former colleague, with whom I've skied and hiked a number of times. He was also in my wedding party over thirty years ago. In addition, the judge for whom I clerked has been a dear friend and ally. I was honored to speak at her wedding, and I always appreciated her speaking at mine. She has told me on a couple of occasions that she regards me as one of her best clerks over her thirty-year career as a judge. I of course appreciated that compliment. It meant something coming from a Stanford grad who was sworn into her judgeship by Supreme Court Justice Sandra Day O'Connor, and who was recognized by the judges on the court as intelligent, driven, and always on top of her caseload.

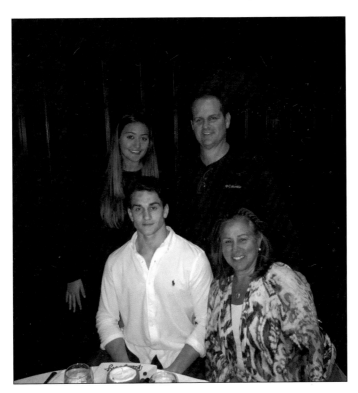

With my family and go-to support group (from left): Taylor, Garrett, and Kim.

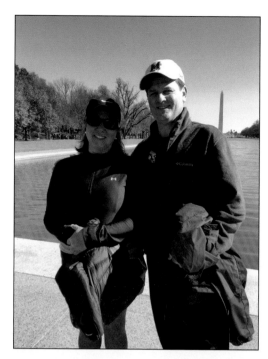

With my best health advocate, Kim, at another cancer fundraiser in Washington, DC.

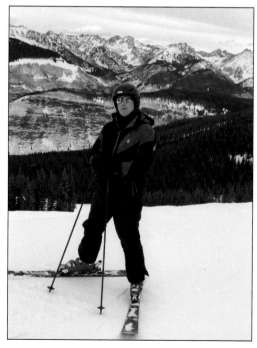

Back on my feet after my first brain surgery—and back on my skis! I haven't tried skiing since my second surgery, but I sure am thinking about taking my son west to ski, now that he has graduated from the University of Maryland. It'll be a bucket list item!

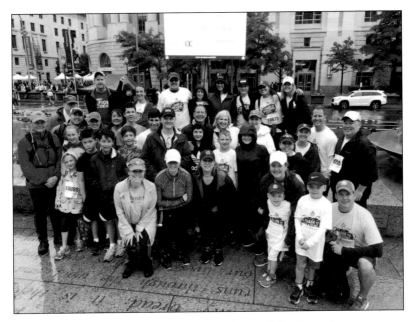

Our team on a rainy-day Race for Hope. Seemed like Race days were always rainy and/or cold. Maybe that kind of weather was appropriate.

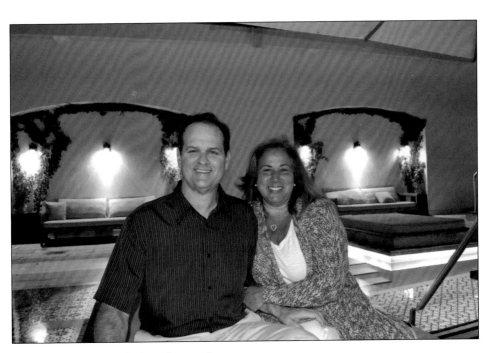

Kim and I enjoying Mexico after my first surgery.

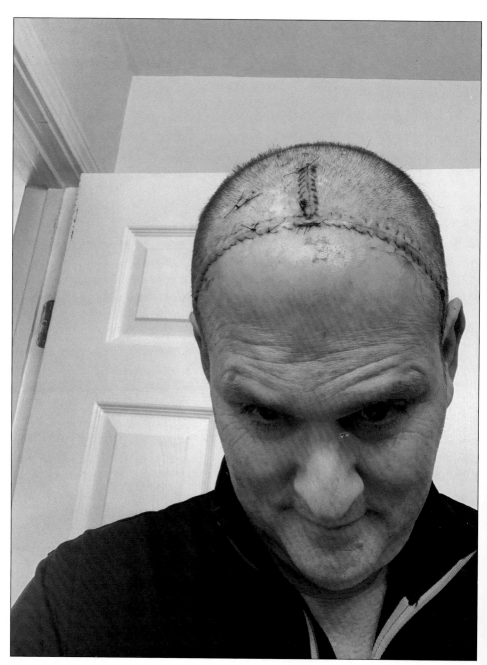

Post-craniotomy: after my second surgery on January 3, 2019.

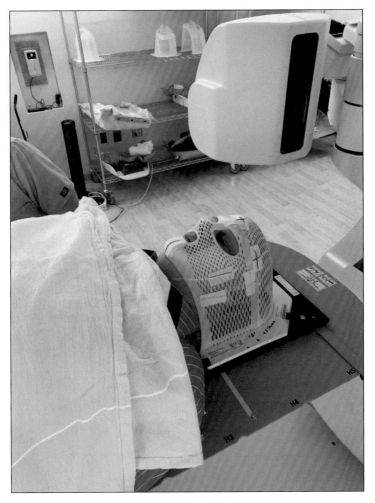

Undergoing radiation treatment at NIH after my second surgery.

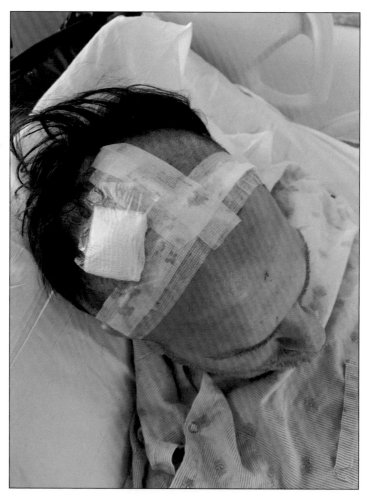

Recovering after my second surgery.

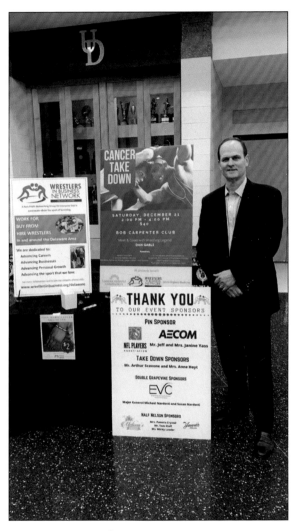

At a wrestling tournament cancer fundraiser event in December 2019 (after my second surgery), I presented at the tournament along with US Senator Chris Coons of Delaware and Olympic Gold Medal wrestler, Dan Gable.

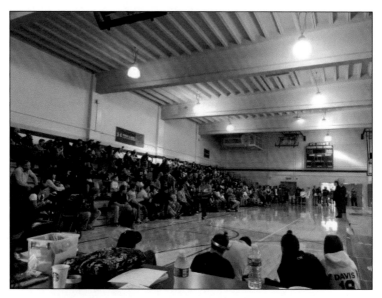

Dr. Henry Brem, the Chief of Neurosurgery at Johns Hopkins Medicine, presenting to the crowd at the fight cancer wrestling tournament organized on my behalf.

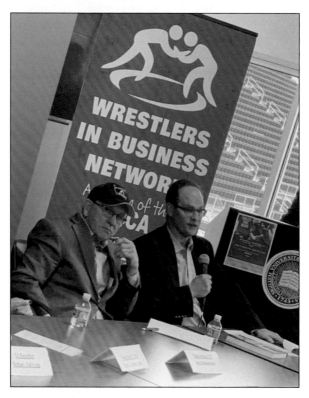

With wrestling legend and Olympic Gold Medalist Dan Gable presenting at a fight cancer program.

Following my judicial clerkship, I went on to work at three top international law firms. I made partner at the first firm reasonably quickly. I was appointed as a practice group leader in a large, highly regarded firm, and then co-chaired a key practice group in another—one of the largest, if not the largest, law firms in the United States. All three of these law firms regularly recruited students from Ivy League and other prestigious law schools.

If I had been assessed solely by objective metrics such as my grades, the steady rise in my legal career would not have been predicted. Fortunately, one's academic background becomes less important as one demonstrates the ability to succeed with cases, to cost-effectively find practical solutions to client problems, and ultimately to develop business.

Other than when I'm trying to market myself for legal work, I rarely discuss my achievements. I mention them here to demonstrate how much I believe all of us can achieve, despite many initial challenges, occasional frustrations, and a lot of failures along the way. I'm proof positive that you can succeed even if you get off to a slow start or you don't take the standard path in life. I believe that once people figure out what really motivates them and where their interests lie, their ability to succeed is unlimited.

I was fortunate to reach the top of my profession reasonably quickly. With success came more difficult challenges. I served as lead counsel on a number of "bet the company" cases involving some of the largest high-profile projects around the world, legal battles where I faced teams of some of the world's top lawyers and experts.

My work has been rich and diverse, generally focused on large-scale construction and infrastructure projects. I served as lead counsel for engineering and construction companies on the Big Dig project in Boston, the Hurricane Katrina recovery project in New Orleans, the Hudson River Tunnel project for the State of New Jersey, the Superstorm Sandy cleanup project in New Jersey, the new Tappan Zee Bridge project, and a number of disputes associated with the Northeast Corridor Rail Improvement Project, involving the Amtrak line between Washington, DC and Boston.

International projects included the multi-billion-dollar Hamad International Airport project in Doha, Qatar. I served as lead counsel for clients such as Discovery Communications and Gucci on their headquarters development projects. A major telecommunications company engaged me on a proposed multi-billion-dollar real estate buildout with IBM of data centers throughout the country.

I found myself in Rio de Janeiro multiple times, representing the international engineering company, AECOM, in connection with the 2016 Olympic Games in Brazil. I also worked with AECOM for many years on major infrastructure projects around the world. Closer to home, and closely aligned with one of my interests, I represented USA Wrestling in the successful effort to bring the sport back into the Olympic Games.

I was appointed by the governor of Maryland to a task force on public-private partnerships and testified side-by-side with the lieutenant governor and the secretary of transportation before the Maryland legislature in support of the law that has become the basis for the massive Purple Line light rail project that is currently underway in Maryland.

Throughout my career, I have published numerous articles in professional journals. John Wiley and Sons (now Aspen

Publishers) published a construction law textbook that I co-authored and edited. I'm proud to have been identified as a top lawyer in the most reputable legal rankings. Despite a slow start and a somewhat unique path through school, toward the end of my thirty-year practice, I was honored to be recognized as an "Eminent Practitioner" in the field of construction law by Chambers and Partners. (Chambers is generally considered the most highly regarded and coveted legal ranking system worldwide.)

None of my achievements could have been foreseen based on my earlier academic performance, or indeed the prestige of the schools from which I graduated. Common wisdom recommends taking the most efficient and effective path in pursuing academic and legal careers: top-of-the-class grade point average leading to acceptance at top universities. That's the traditional course, and that's what many people seek. Had I thought it would work for me, I may very well have taken that more traditional approach—although I hesitate to say that's a definite. I just was not a big fan of studying back in my high school and college days. Unfortunately, I just wasn't passionate enough about school to work hard enough to achieve the top grades.

As it turns out, following an unconventional path was the best fit for me. I believe this path may be appropriate for others as well—for those who might not be successful on the more conventional path, or who feel the conventional way is just not right for them. By and large, this approach may make sense for many professions, not just law. Different people have different personalities and preferences, and they need to find the path and the approaches that best suit them.

I ultimately found that I had developed a strong interest in the practical side of legal work and business. As I was exposed more to legal work in different contexts, I grew more confident in my ability to succeed in the profession. Success breeds confidence, and confidence breeds success.

I gained a better appreciation for the fairly basic notion in the legal profession: Clients are paying real money and want their problems solved cost-effectively. For clients, it's really about getting a problem solved for a reasonable price. In the end, clients are paying for results. And I was finally facing real-life problems where the results mattered to my clients.

So my goal was straightforward: to be an effective advocate on behalf of clients. My competitive side, honed earlier via participation in sports in general and particularly in the one-on-one aspects of wrestling, helped drive my desire to be a successful lawyer.

I never sought to achieve results that I didn't feel were appropriate for my clients. Indeed, if I thought my clients' goals for a case were unreasonable or unrealistic, or that they did not have a persuasive case, I would tell them up front that they would need to dial back their expectations. Sometimes we had to rethink the case and how we would proceed. This may have limited my work at times and impacted my fees, but I was okay with that, since it really was the right approach. Giving clients the best possible advice was, and had to be, more important than generating fees. I always felt that fees would follow from other cases that had more merit.

Perhaps the unconventional path I took in my earlier years taught me the importance of greater persistence, diligence, and resilience in overcoming difficult problems. It also taught me that I was always going to have to prove myself to succeed. I'd like to think that the strength I gained by being more persistent over the years helped me to fight through and survive my health crisis.

As my career evolved, the approach I tried to take had more simplicity to it than magic. Maybe most successful people take a similar tack. I've learned to isolate the problem from everything else that is occurring, weigh all the competing considerations, and then try to pursue the most effective solution. I'd focus on the most pressing and important issues, so that other competing issues were essentially put on hold. The many construction projects I dealt with were large and complex, with many variables.

Isolate the problem, weigh the options, figure out a solution, and pursue it. Like everything else worth achieving, this simple, isolate-weigh-pursue approach takes practice. It's not lost on me that it's easier said than done. And in law, things become a little more challenging, as you're generally working in the context of a client budget and dealing with a problem that the client couldn't solve itself. You may have to pass over certain issues due to financial constraints. Part of the critical thinking, and maybe it's part of the art required for successful law practice, involves determining which issues to focus on for a given case and which issues likely will not impact the final result.

Fortunately, I have found that when one challenges an obstacle with critical thinking, the right focus, and determined effort, one can persevere and succeed. There is never a need to give up on reasonably achievable goals for which one is passionate. One should never doubt one's capabilities, and there is no room for excuses on the path to accomplishment.

My successes in life have corresponded with my definite share of failures. When I failed, it usually was because I wasn't focusing on the most relevant issues. As I grew older, the path to

success seemed to become clearer. Achieving success in address-
ing a complex issue requires a mature and clear understanding
of the situation, an organized approach, hard work, sacrifice,
dedication, creative and practical thinking, and good old-fash-
ioned common sense. I've also found that success is best and
most effectively achieved by acting at all times with character
and integrity. While these may seem like unremarkable traits,
one should never lose sight of their importance and how they
can contribute to one's happiness and sense of accomplishment.

In addition, it never hurts to pursue one's goals with a sense
of humor and thoughtful optimism. I've always tried to maintain
a pleasant personality, a sound demeanor, and a good sense of
humor, even in difficult situations. Additionally, as I've grown
older and matured, I've never felt comfortable unless I stayed
driven, determined, and effective. My aim was sharpened by
seeking to achieve something of value for my clients.

To sum up: A slow start need not prevent a strong finish.
Becoming an effective advocate for the interests of stakeholders
is a vital element of success. Developing an isolate-weigh-pursue
approach to problems is also vital, as are such basic virtues as
honesty, hard work, and an optimistic attitude. Combine these
and other elements I've explored, and I believe you have a recipe
for achievement.

As something of a sanity check, as the final edits to my book
were being completed, I ran across an article by the legendary
Warren Buffett on how kids should think about their passions.
Buffett said:

Whether you define success in terms of finances, or professional achievement, or art, or invention—or even just

growing up to be an honorable, trustworthy person—this all comes down to two sides of the same coin:

1. Encourage young people to explore broadly and embrace the things that speak to their interests, passions—and yes, their eccentricities.

2. But also encourage them to learn how the world works; don't blindly follow your passions, but instead learn to find things that work in practice, and narrow your possible pursuits down to the few among them that can inspire your passions.

Chapter Fourteen
Work, Wealth, Health, and Friendship

A good friend of mine told me that his company wanted him to assume a new position late in his career. He was just a couple years away from retirement, and his boss wanted him to take on a managerial position. For the first time in his career, he would be in charge of a number of employees, leading group meetings, and potentially firing those who were not performing well.

Understandably, my friend felt that in taking on the new role, his success would no longer be dependent solely on his own work, but rather on how successful his employees were. The situation represented a brand-new source of stress for him.

As we discussed his situation, my friend invoked the old expression, usually credited to Friedrich Nietzsche: "What doesn't kill you makes you stronger."

Even though I am living proof of someone who was incredibly weakened by an illness that did not manage to kill me, I still manage to appreciate the truth contained in those words. Surely people won't grow if they aren't pushing themselves to the next level of pressure. As they say, "No pressure, no diamonds." I understand that one's success with more difficult tasks may give one the strength to take on even greater responsibilities.

But my friend got me thinking about the phrase. It could be the case that the more stressful the task one is assigned, the greater the toll it is taking on one's life. A corollary expression could be: what doesn't kill you isn't necessarily helping you. The pressure might actually be causing you harm, with negative impacts to your health of which you're not even aware.

Especially as you get older, what doesn't kill you just may wind up hurting you. To avoid the harmful effects of stress, it's important to exercise regularly, get annual physicals, and have stress tests or other assessments that show the effects of stress. Sometimes a stressful job just might not be the best thing for you.

Some people thrive and grow under pressure. For others, it has a toxic impact. Specifically, many people cannot handle the stress of managing people. Yet others generate strength from taking on managerial roles.

Perhaps the stress of my legal work took a hidden toll on me physically. In my professional life, I was responsible for the success of a number of partners and associates in my firms. Perhaps I wasn't fully appreciating the impact that my managerial role was having on my health.

As a younger associate starting out in law and attempting to move up in the ranks, it seemed important to me to work hard in my law firms so that I could make partner. Making partner in a major law firm was essentially the brass ring that almost all associates wanted to achieve. In private practice, for many it's a sign of success if you're elected to the partnership at a large, well-respected law firm. Maybe it's a sign that you're "not quite cutting it" if you don't make partner. The positive side is you've learned that you need to rethink your work priorities.

From my new-found, post-operative perspective, I suppose I have to challenge my old assumptions a bit. Is making partner in a major firm really that important? In a financial sense, partnership is important, as one needs to pay for one's home and food, and raise and take care of a family: so indeed partnership helps pay the bills. Generally, though, what you want is a good, solid core of satisfied clients for whom you're consistently generating positive results. I suspect that one can achieve excellent results for clients whether or not one ever becomes a partner in a major firm. Perhaps there is an exception here to the "larger is better" rule of thumb.

Early on in my legal practice, it became clear that many of the best and larger clients with the most complex legal issues ended up retaining major law firms. Boards of directors of major companies feel compelled to hire the top, well-known law firms. As a general matter, hiring larger, well-respected firms can never be criticized by the board of directors or shareholders of companies. That's just the way the world seems to work. Perhaps this is one of the reasons positions in larger firms are more attractive to young lawyers. Also, the larger firms have a higher salary range and clients that can pay the sizable bills that major law firms tend to generate on complex matters.

But for many, the success of partnership comes at a price. In the end, in major firms, if you make partner, there is a lot of pressure to generate substantial amounts of business from major clients. Once you've been a partner for a number of years at a major law firm, the expectation is that you're an excellent lawyer. Your proficiency as a lawyer is simply expected once you've made partner.

While I was very proud to be elected to the partnership in three major law firms and served in leadership as a chair or co-chair in these firms, perhaps it came at a price that affected my health. I don't know. Was I really achieving a valuable purpose? I'm sure I felt that way at the time. I was making the firm more profitable, and it was my job to do that. However, maybe I paid the price in terms of my health? I hope not, but I'll never know.

Of course, it was important that I was able to support my family. So far, I've been able to raise my children to be productive individuals with solid values. The law firms for whom I've worked have given me the financial wherewithal to do that. So, in that respect, I served a purpose beyond simply improving the law firm's bottom line. Hopefully, I've also set a good example for my children.

A common thread that runs through my whole life is to try to make things better. It's a mindset based on my belief in hope and progress.

"Why are you always trying to change things!" my family and friends would often respond in reaction to this or that attempt on my part to establish a more effective, positive, or rational approach to a given situation. My goal has always been to make things better for everyone. I would never suggest change simply for the sake of change. My goal was never to disrupt a process that was working reasonably well.

A somewhat humorous example of where I tried to improve things: a friend asked me to do a reading at his wedding. It was an ancient poem. Before I read the poem at his wedding, I decided to make a couple tweaks of my own to it. After the wedding ceremony, my friend asked me quizzically with a grin on his face: "Did you change the poem?"

"Sure," I responded. "Didn't it sound better?"

My friend shook his head and laughed. "Come to think of it, you did make it sound better."

I see myself as a friendly and outgoing guy. I always enjoy connecting with people. I have friends from every phase of my life, from school, from my law career, from sports teams, and from my children's busy lives. I used to give Garrett and Taylor a simple piece of advice: In whatever stage of life you find yourselves, you'll probably end up with three or four close relationships. Every school, every sorority or fraternity, every extracurricular activity—you'll probably find three or four people with whom you'll form strong friendships and with whom you see eye to eye and trust on issues. These people will serve as a mutual support network later in life. You may be surrounded by hundreds, even thousands of fellow students at school, but don't expect to have thirty or forty friends. That's just not realistic—at least not for me. You'll probably end up with other acquaintances and contacts. They may never become close friends, but it's nice to know they're out there.

Developing several solid friendships from all stages of my life is the way things progressed for me. First and foremost, I genuinely like these people. I suspect that my approach on forming relationships is not all that novel. I've really found it valuable to develop these friendships every step of the way.

After being hit with a brain tumor and the follow-up treatments, I saw my role in life change in very definite ways. For my children and for the benefit of others, I want to look for ways to serve a valuable purpose in life. I believe parents and others should still feel very satisfied with their lives if they've successfully managed to raise their children or the next generation to be solid, upstanding, and contributing citizens. However, my health situation has motivated me to pursue a further goal.

I've decided that my focus should be on a new and important purpose: to help support the fight against brain cancer. It's an obligation I feel I need to fulfill and support. I plan to continue to do fundraising and see that those funds are actually used in a meaningful way.

Another part of my effort to serve the greater good is to complete this book, which I hope will be helpful to other people who find themselves in the midst of challenges, medical or otherwise. I write about my experience in this book to offer my thoughts on approaching, and even triumphing, in the face of tremendous adversity.

The actual work of writing is far more of a time-consuming effort than it used to be. The unpredictable workings of my brain can cause what I'll call "the puzzle pieces" to change shape mid-puzzle. Yet I still prefer writing over the actual puzzles my occupational therapists would ask me to solve, or the tasks that they would assign me, like reading a menu and ordering fictitious meals within a certain budget or sending me around the rehabilitation hospital on a scavenger hunt of sorts.

I'm no longer practicing law. Nevertheless, I'm actually trying to enjoy this new stage of life. I'm passionate about engaging in activities that serve a higher purpose, that help other people and have a positive impact on a wider community than just myself, my clients, and my family. It's taken years, but I see the pursuit of my current goals as an escape from more troubling thoughts, as well as a healthy way to challenge my brain.

Chapter Fifteen

Finding Happiness within a "New Normal"

Where I am right now is the proverbial "new normal," and it's a place I never thought I'd end up during the hustle and bustle of my legal career.

With the tumor still in my brain, and given what I've been through, I conduct a minor ritual after waking up each morning, in the middle of the night, or after daily naps. I methodically assess my balance, brain function, speech, dizziness, and basic functioning. I do this during or after most any activity, including something as seemingly simple as conducting a one-on-one conversation.

The results of these quick checks are rarely perfect. My condition is flawed in many ways that would not be obvious to most people and seem to differ at various times of the day or evening for reasons I can't explain. But the inexplicable changes do make me wonder what's really going on "up there."

Even for something as simple as taking a daily shower, getting dressed, or even just getting coffee, I tend to follow a routine of sorts. In essence it's my own effort to practice mindfulness, but in connection with my daily needs in life. It gives me some sense of control. I find it mentally refreshing to follow a routine in these seemingly mundane contexts. Have I done these basic tasks in life in the most logical order? Again, it sounds a bit like my apparent preference for real life activities over hypotheticals. It's also become my own daily check on operations upstairs.

My version of mindfulness also involves self-questioning. How will I handle things that I used to just take for granted? Will my next MRI lead to favorable results? My wife and I celebrate things that would never cross the minds of most people. That is, when I get my MRI results back and there is no finding of tumor growth, we couldn't be happier.

This constant level of self-observance and personal celebration feels a bit surreal. I certainly notice flaws more than a common observer likely would. I work hard to try to keep my deficits in check so they really are not obvious to anyone but me. Except in the eyes of a barber, the scars on my head from my surgeries barely show. I need to nap far more frequently, but no one sees that except for my family.

I've found that when I look and act fairly normally—which I can generally pull off—most people, even close family and friends, will have difficulty comprehending or appreciating how I feel both mentally and physically. I can almost hear their inner comments:

"Hey, Bob, you look pretty good. Why don't you just do all the same things you used to?"

I wish. It takes some effort to rise to the occasion. When I engage in social activities, I approach them differently and for shorter periods. I gravitate to quieter areas and speak less. While these activities may not be the best fit for me and quickly tire me out, I try to do them when it's the right thing to do. Generally I am able to manage relationships reasonably well, but for shorter periods of time.

While I have to deal with these issues, and don't like making accommodations, I have no choice. I'd rather not have to explain myself. I think it's hard for most people to appreciate that a meal, discussion, or walk, during which I looked pretty good, will require that I retreat to a quiet location to get some sleep and rebuild my mental strength and my ability to concentrate. I enjoyed many years of endless hours doing complex legal work with boundless energy. Now my mind operates like an aging cell phone, one where the battery runs down quickly and needs frequent recharges.

As of 2020, I'm now facing a couple of other adverse impacts of my treatment that are making my life a little too interesting. A new and unexpected change for me (apparently quite unusual) has been my need to rely on my right eye a little more as my left optic nerve and vision suffered some slight damage during my radiation therapy.

Yet another curve ball: my MRI of October 7, 2020, showed an unusual change which the MRI report identified as potential tumor growth. The MRI report is now being examined by six of the nation's top doctors at Johns Hopkins, UCSF, and NIH. The MRI report and growth are also being reviewed by the tumor board at Hopkins. Hopefully, the growth is radiation damage, but no one can tell us definitively. We just have to hope that my next MRI (now accelerated) will show stability in this growth.

I'm not planning to "shuffle off this mortal coil" anytime soon, and I give my family that reassurance all the time. I would never let my current challenges do me in. In fact, the existence of these difficulties reminds me of how fortunate I am to have made it through the worst of medical experiences. My miracle—I am still here, but there's never a dull moment.

I've found that I can't concentrate like I used to, take in details, focus, or read anything for a long period of time. Speaking has become a challenge due to the impact on the coordination of my tongue movement impacted by my cerebellum bleed, and speaking clearly and projecting my voice has become quite tiring. I've found it's best for me to speak at close range and in quieter areas. That my computer reads back my writing has been a life saver in terms of concentrating for this writing. My primary goal is to get this story out and to offer help wherever it might be well-received. I hope to provide both perspective and appreciation for what has worked for me, what hasn't, and what I believe can work for others. Again, I try to stay fairly modest, because while I believe that I've accomplished some good things, I also believe that there is more that I can do.

At any stage in life, when one finds the need to take an alternative path, perhaps others will point out the obstacles involved. However, I didn't really see the path I took as presenting serious problems. To the contrary, for me, adversity presented interesting challenges that ultimately had a positive outcome. The challenges caused me to develop a better appreciation for the importance of diligence, perseverance, and finding passion in all aspects of life. Throughout my life, I've had a tendency to do things a bit differently from others. I haven't done this simply for the sake of being different. While I haven't always been right, I've always felt that the path I chose made sense and was reasonable and logical for me.

The clarity I ultimately gained came at a price that no one

should ever have to pay. While I faced—and continue to face—the difficulties of a brain tumor and the damage caused by the stroke and other problems, the silver lining is that these issues caused me to reflect on and find a better perspective on some important aspects of life, including academic and career paths, capitalizing on strengths, persevering through weaknesses, and finding your passion. I am better able to connect the proverbial dots that we sometimes miss when confronting our challenges.

As my health crisis has progressed, I've spoken to many different people and thought about a lot of different aspects of my experience. To achieve my goals, obviously I need to do everything reasonably possible to stay alive. I want to lead a full life and feel as though my time here on earth has had meaning and purpose.

Fortunately, I've done a lot of things which really do make me feel as though I've lived life fully. I've done a lot to raise my children the right way and feel motivated to see them succeed in their careers, become happily married, and have children of their own—as in our grandchildren.

I know Kim and I will enjoy grandparenting. While I will be thinking about my mortality with some frequency, I remain open to miracles and truly grateful for all the rewards of my life. There's still a lot more to do and live for. And as I always remind myself, it's not where you start, but where you finish.

PART THREE

Examining Your Life: Twelve Essays

It's a sobering business, this staring down the fact of our own mortality. I can tell from experience that it tends to focus the mind tremendously. Distracting thoughts get burned away. Trivialities disappear. What is really important is thrown into sharp relief. I discovered a somewhat odd but very comforting truth: in thinking about my mortality, my mind concentrates not on death, but on life, and how to live it well.

What follows are twelve meditations of a sort, or essays if you will, on subjects that I find myself centering in on, ever since the idea that I would someday die suddenly exploded from the theoretical to the real, from the abstract to the concrete. The religious leader Martin Luther tacked up his famous "Ninety-Five Theses" on a church door in Wittenberg, Germany. These are a dozen mini-essays that I am nailing to the door.

1. Don't Expect Life to Proceed as Planned

"Man makes plans and God laughs." That ancient piece of wisdom reminds us that life is full of surprise twists and sharp, abrupt turns.

I don't have to look too far in my own experience to discover the truth of this cautionary rule of thumb. My family was deep into planning our vacation to Mexico, reserving the flight, confirming our hotel, and thinking about a range of fun activities. Then God gave a snort of laughter at our plans and wiped them all away abruptly when doctors diagnosed me with brain cancer.

Generally, human beings don't like surprises. Or rather they enjoy tidy, easily manageable surprises—reassuring ones that indicate they're flexible and not easily upset. An unexpected birthday gift might be an acceptable exception to the general "no surprises" rule. But even there, the surprise party is a notoriously iffy shock to spring on anyone near and dear. (Most of us say we wouldn't want one, and though some of us might be fibbing, surveys tell us that three out of five people sincerely don't want one.)

When our lives don't follow a predictable course, there's a double danger. The first is that we have to change our plans or expectations, and the second is that we have to deal with our anger, hurt, or frustration at the sudden shift in fortunes: How on earth could heaven do this to me?

As a matter of human nature, we end up harming ourselves

by persisting in useless resistance or protest. Such a reaction is understandable, but ultimately useless. It simply does no good. Go along with a change of fortune, face it square on, and deal with it.

For reasons of circumstance or personality, when I was diagnosed with cancer I didn't waste time bewailing my fate. Somehow I intuitively understood that my best move was to think of ways I could meet the new challenge most effectively. That was the direction I saw as most productive. Don't get me wrong; I definitely went through a stage of shock and disbelief when I first got the diagnosis. But I then moved reasonably quickly into a more productive, thoughtful, and solutions-oriented mode.

I might have developed a disciplined response to adversity during my time wrestling and in other competitive periods of my life. In the high school version of the sport, matches are six minutes long. That means split-second decisions and lightning-fast reactions. There is no time to fuss over reversals. In wrestling, your goal is to get to the point where you "break" your opponents—that is, you want your opponents to feel like they are going to lose.

Sure, I made plans before each match and thought through strategies I felt might work against a given opponent. I would speak with my coach and we considered moves that might succeed. But I wouldn't get fixated on any move. In the heat of battle, it was important to remain flexible to adapt to a constantly changing match. Wrestling taught me not to get too attached to something that's not working. If a half nelson failed, be ready to switch to a tight waist followed by an arm bar.

Relevant here are the wise words of General Norman

Schwarzkopf: "A plan is always the first casualty of war." We know this to be true, our experience tells us as much, yet again and again we ignore this wisdom and stick stubbornly to our plans. We are like gamblers who fall victim to the "sunk value" fallacy: they are on a losing streak, but they throw good money after bad in the vain hope their luck will change.

My time spent on the wrestling mat in high school and college and watching my son in the sport left me with indelible patterns of behavior that I took forward into my legal career and into my life in general. Even when I lost a match, I was learning. We all know about the impatience of a child who wishes for a present six months before a birthday. With time, the child grows up and, with luck, learns the lesson of persistence and fortitude.

It's good to remind parents that all that time spent in the bleachers was not in vain, watching while their children dropped one match after another. The sport definitely generates anxiety. The kids involved might have been on the losing end of things in the short run, but they were picking up valuable lessons that they will carry with them their whole lives. They might acquire the attitude of the joy of competition and seeing which moves worked and which did not. Greater flexibility comes with maturity and developing the kind of "muscle memory" that leads to a quick response in a given situation.

Every reversal, every time a change of plans is forced upon us, there's always some emotional pain involved. Our impulse is to grieve over what might have been. Most of us have heard about the five stages of grief: denial, anger, bargaining, depression, and acceptance. My attitude has always been a bit different. How about I skip over one through four, I tell myself, and land on the acceptance part right off the bat?

Lately I've heard about another stage of that process, one more action to add to the other five: Gratitude. To see death or an ending as an aspect of something so large, so wonderful, that the negative aspects get swallowed up by thankfulness. I can't always accomplish such a high-minded trick, but it's something I can aspire to.

Yes, life serves up curve balls. I was serving on a three-person arbitration panel assisting in deciding a case right at the time when I was diagnosed with a brain tumor. I had to leave the panel to deal with my health crisis. I was replaced as a panelist by another lawyer, who I heard later passed away out of the blue due to heart complications. The chairperson of the panel also passed from a disease he had been fighting for quite a while. Then a law partner of mine died in his sleep on New Year's Eve, of all times.

I pondered these developments with a mix of sadness and shock. It didn't make any sense. I was the one with cancer, yet all these colleagues had passed away ahead of me. I was left mourning their loss and marveling at the quirks of fate. The moral I took away from that experience was to keep moving forward with life. It just might not be your turn.

Keep planning, in other words, but be ready to adapt. Who knows? Things could break your way. That family vacation I had had to give up? I wound up going with the family two years later than originally scheduled. We enjoyed ourselves all the more knowing we had dodged a bullet a couple of years earlier.

What plans have you been forced to change or give up due to altered circumstances?

2. What's Really Important

Life's not easy for any of us. Day-to-day living at times requires us to scramble around, rushing from one minor crisis to another. The writer Jack Kerouac talked about "urgencies, false and otherwise," and those are what we feel we have to answer to.

That's how I lived my life for a long time. I flew all over the world, attending to other people's issues, getting to "yes," and arriving at the right solution. I always had a lot of balls in the air. I actually enjoyed the sense of being busy. I'm a competitive person, and each fork in the road offered me a chance to choose the winning route.

But what happened when I got hit with a cancer diagnosis? Suddenly my perspective shifted. The old truths didn't seem to be true any longer. I found myself challenging all my assumptions and questioning my home truths.

It doesn't have to be cancer. It could be any life-altering, "before-and-after" event. The death of a loved one. A natural disaster. Trouble with a relationship you believed was rock solid. The point is, when something of this magnitude occurs, the rug is pulled out from under you. In fact, sometimes the floor underneath the rug falls away, too. You find yourself in free fall.

That happened to me. What previously seemed vitally important, now appeared trivial or easily dismissed. The terms of my contract with life got rewritten. I always believed that I could handle the stress of a high-level legal career. Now I questioned that. Could the life I had been leading hurt me in some way? Had it somehow left me open for serious illness?

More than that, more than questions about my old realities, I also discovered a yearning, a real hunger, and a pressing demand for new answers. It came down to asking a basic question. What is really important to me?

I had been on the treadmill—the hamster wheel—of my career. Now I had a chance to pull the cord and step off. I had suffered a "catastrophic loss." I was deemed totally disabled. No one had any right to expect anything of me beyond vegetable status.

The poet Robert Frost stated that he knew one thing for certain about life: "It goes on." After two brain surgeries I was overjoyed to discover that I was still capable of thought, action, and emotion. My life went on. And I had a new goal: to reformulate what was important in my life.

It wasn't anything new, really—it was more a case of retrieving and revitalizing something that had gotten lost in the scramble of everyday life. I had been afflicted with such a narrow focus that I tended to lose sight of the big picture.

What was the big picture? Well, I knew it had to do with being a solid and honorable person and doing the right thing. When I meditated on this, the simple word that floated up in my mind was "helping." Given my circumstance, helping meant putting my efforts toward helping to find a cure for cancer. When I asked myself what was important, what was meaningful, the answer came back loud and clear: Put my shoulder to the wheel. Throw myself into a new and more meaningful life.

On a selfish, day-to-day basis, I wanted to extend my own life. But beyond that, beyond the small picture, I wanted to be a part of something much bigger. Many, many people around the world work toward curing cancer. In order to contribute, I stand upon the shoulders of giants who have already made enormous progress.

Religion and philosophy are all about asking what is meaningful in life. They remind us to put the treadmill of life on pause. Being a good person, doing the right thing, helping others—these are basic values all over the world. These values ask us to look beyond ourselves.

Though I realize they are vital to many people, the rituals of religion seem less necessary to me than the underlying message. I prefer thought-provoking services, with folks talking about meaningful subjects. I like to be reminded of the big picture in ways that I may not have considered on my own.

Whenever I asked myself what was really important to me, I found I kept returning again and again to my children. And I realized that part of the big picture involves taking the long view. I was looking down the road to my children's adult lives, and beyond that, to the lives of their children and their children's children.

The treadmill life demanded that I concentrate on the next minute, the next lap, the next iteration. The focus was right at the end of my nose. But once I shifted away from that perspective, I realized how myopic it is. Once in a while, I now tell myself, I have to raise my eyes beyond the immediate future and take the long view.

I sent a list of these essay subjects out to a few of my friends to get their comments. "I realize that I'm violating, like, ten of your principles," one person responded. He was deep in mid-career.

I laughed, telling him he was free to ignore any or all of them. "Otherwise you'll go broke," I said, both of us laughing. Despite our laugh over this, I believe there's minimal to no cost in following the guidance I offered in any of these issues. And maybe that "no cost" factor is the real blessing.

No one can focus on the meaningful and important constantly. If you devote yourself exclusively to taking in the big picture all the time, you're liable to trip over an obstacle lying right at your feet. But I remind myself that once in a while—not always, not every minute of every day, but every so often—I have to remember what's truly important in life.

What's really important to you? Do you have the right long view?

3. Achieve Greater Peace by Controlling What Really Matters

I recently had a morning where two of my family members were tugging at me from different directions, and it made me think about the difference between things I can and can't control. My daughter announced she and her boyfriend were going to stay in an Airbnb rental in nearby Baltimore to attend a Halloween party at a nearby bar. And my wife wanted to speak to me about her ideas for remodeling the kitchen.

I said to Taylor: "It's stupid for you to go to a party right now with the pandemic raging." I'm the furthest thing from a kill-joy, but this party sounded like a super-spreader event in the making. I am medically vulnerable to viruses, and a COVID infection could have a potential lethal impact.

But Taylor was of an age that I felt I could no longer make choices for her. She is typically quite careful and knows when a situation carries a risk. I can only give my opinion on a subject and hope she would see it my way. She agreed that, when she returned from the party, she would quarantine away from us, get tested, and make sure we stayed clear of each other until we were confident she was COVID-free.

As for remodeling the kitchen, that was a bridge too far for me. I told Kim that I really didn't want to stretch myself to think about kitchen remodeling. The countless decisions in décor, design, and layout sounded like too many stressors from a realm that was just not important enough to be worth the worry. We also had many other home improvement projects that we had yet to put a dent in.

More and more, I try to make decisions by weighing the amount of anxiety they are going to cause. I see it as a method of decluttering my life and my mind. The popular author and lifestyle expert Marie Kondo triggered a whole movement focused on physically tidying up one's domestic surroundings. Rearranging your interior life—tidying up your mental clutter— is a parallel and just as vital an enterprise. I want to concentrate on two areas that are of paramount importance to me: staying healthy and helping as much as I can in the fight against cancer. In order to be able to do this, I have to clear out as many distractions as possible.

No one is getting out of this world alive. I recall a TED talk I listened to years ago from a gentleman who had been given a limited time to live by his doctors. (I watched this video long before I was diagnosed with a brain tumor.) The talk triggered a lot of TED-style questions of my own. How could this gentleman speak with such composure and how could he be so reflective knowing he didn't have long to live? Could I deal with his situation with the same level of equanimity, and how would I accomplish that?

I didn't give it a lot of thought back then, as my life was not immediately at risk. Now that I'm faced with a life-threatening disease, I've thought about the subject much more. I've concluded that my composure would depend on the degree to which I felt I had my affairs in order. First and foremost that meant ensuring that my family was financially secure and otherwise ready to succeed in the real world. If I had those aspects of my life under control, I decided, I would be able to face with confidence whatever was thrown at me.

Lately I've returned to that idea with a new level of focus. I think I see it as the foundational stage of security. My children have proceeded along the college and graduate school paths and have succeeded well enough that I'm confident I've established a foundational beginning to their lives. Everything beyond the foundational stage, including things like getting married and having children of their own, are not yet pressing issues. However, I feel that I instilled good judgment in my children to properly handle their next stages in life. And I knew Kim would still be around to guide them and to celebrate as they proceeded through all the great things life has to offer.

Decluttering my life so I can better concentrate on my main goals involves making choices. I will care about *this* (protecting myself from illness), and I don't want to spend my time thinking about *that* (remodeling the kitchen). And I really didn't think any kitchen remodeling was needed.

My family tells me they believe my personality has changed. Maybe it has. Maybe I'm just getting closer to what my true personality was all along, before I began being bombarded with countless work and schedule demands. Frankly, if my personality has evolved, I'm hoping the "new me" is a better version of myself, especially when compared to my former work-encumbered personality.

It's true that life can be seen as the tension between what you want to do and what others want you to do. Just the other day, I mentioned that I really didn't want to haul suitcases down our stairway. The kids could do that. Past experience has shown me that carrying heavy suitcases down the stairs has definitely hurt my back.

"Dad!" the kids exclaimed. "Can you help us for once?" I saw this "help us for once" comment as a bit of challenge to which I really shouldn't have to answer. I'm not a complainer, but I've been beaten up quite a bit medically for years. Maybe I felt as though I should be cut some slack.

I knew that, for years, I had done an awful lot to help the kids with school, examining career directions, and finding jobs. I still help in this vitally important area. I've also always helped around the house, supported the family, and created a nice lifestyle for them.

A little troubled by my kids' comments, I began thinking that the money didn't grow on trees for mortgages, tuitions, food on the table, and for virtually all the family's expenses. I also did many things behind the scenes to contribute to our household running smoothly.

Thinking it through though, I began to realize that I was just never going to win this debate and it wasn't worth the argument. I suspect they'll figure it out one day when they're older and have kids of their own.

Simplify and get the clutter out of your life. There are all sorts of areas in my life where I can streamline things. For example, monitoring my use of the internet and other exposure to media helped to get rid of a lot of stress, leading to a greater sense of calmness and comfort. I realized I didn't need to know every new development, every turn of the news cycle, and every rotation of the globe. I've taken greater control of what I see and hear. I still listen to news reports here and there, just enough to know that we haven't come under nuclear attack, and that I can continue dealing with what I feel is truly important in my life.

Technology is a mixed blessing. I really own very few devices that feature alarms, notifications, random beeps, and ringtones. Watches that talk, screens that flash, units that respond by robotic voice—I see the whole modern array of devices as unnecessary. Or, I see each device in my life as something that is likely to break. I also feel that I survived in the world just fine without these devices. But, I will concede that I could see the value in some of the heart health information relayed by certain smart phone apps.

A friend with whom I do a lot of walking for exercise asked, "Do you have a Fitbit or something like that to keep track of your steps?"

"Nah," I said. I don't keep track of how many steps I take in a day. I just walk and generally know the distance of my walk. I don't care if I finish ten seconds faster or slower on any given day. The real point is to make sure I get regular exercise. Having to check my time, distance, or number of steps represents just one more thought that I can eliminate, one more worry that would distract from my day-to-day existence.

There is a large box in the guest room of our home that has remained sitting in the same place since my birthday well over a year ago. It contains a new large hanging foyer light that Kim felt we needed. In a past period of my life, I would let that box nag at me until I did something about it. I would have put the lamp together and gotten it hung.

Lately I just breeze past the sitting box and other minor demands on my time. There's window work, electrical work, drywall work, and painting to be done. Paint color is the first thing that needs to be determined. Well, paint color is Kim's department. Do I think about these undone tasks? Not nearly as much as I used to. It's a better and less stressful way to live.

I don't want to suggest that I am now this lofty, important person who has more meaningful things to do than attend to the minutiae of existence. That's not it at all. I just believe we can all take greater control of what we allow to control us. The modern world demands our attention in all sorts of ways. I've learned to develop strategies to pick and choose what kind of demands I'll tend to.

A crucible is a fire that burns away impurities to leave what's valuable behind. There is a metallurgic meaning of the word, and also a metaphorical one: a situation of severe trial which leads to the creation of something new. Cancer served as my crucible. It helped me to determine what was truly valuable and necessary.

What do you consider truly valuable and necessary in your life?

4. What's My Prognosis?

When I was diagnosed with a brain tumor, I wanted to get a better understanding of my cancer and what it would mean for me. I did what everyone does and what physicians hate, which was that I tried to find answers on my own.

I googled my disease.

With seventeen innocent taps on a computer keyboard, I spelled out "oligodendroglioma" in the search box. My browser gave me several more search choices even though I wasn't probing for them. Among them was "oligodendroglioma prognosis." Given my understanding of the risks associated with computer searches for complex issues, I was reluctant to see what a click on that choice might yield. But I felt like I had to take a look. I remember a question running through my mind. What would it tell me? I thought that maybe it would give me twenty years to live.

I couldn't resist. I clicked "oligodendroglioma prognosis." The results altered my thinking about my health forever.

A diagnosis is a statement of the present. A prognosis, on the other hand, is a look into the crystal ball of the future. The members of my medical team were fairly certain of their diagnosis. I had a kind of brain cancer that manifested itself in a rare kind of tumor. Their prognosis was positive, but still a bit vague. They spoke in generalities, or somewhat inexact time frames. It felt like the home service providers, who give you only a window of time for when the technician might show up at your house. "The cable guy will be there some time between two o'clock and five."

In contrast to my physicians, the internet laid it right on the line: "People with grade III oligodendrogliomas are expected to live an average of three-point-five years." That was a startling thing to read. I'm thinking about twenty years to live and the search gives me only three-and-a-half? Really? What could that mean? I speculated—the best I could expect was five or six years?

Those dozen or so words put my situation in stark terms. I saw it as establishing something of a deadline for my mortality. As long as I live, I suspect I will never be without the thought of three-and-a-half years or so as a limit for my time on earth. I reached out to Dr. Lattera, my oncologist, and mentioned the Google prognosis.

"Well, no," he responded. "With chemotherapy and radiation, we are currently talking in terms of ten years before we'll see any additional growth in your tumor."

In giving his prognosis, Dr. Laterra was referring not to death but to additional tumor enhancement or growth. Wisely, I've chosen to rely on my neuro-oncologist at Hopkins, but I must say the terms spelled out in black and white on the internet do linger in my mind.

On the all-important goal of staying alive, my doctors have never given me a prognosis consistent with the results of my computer search. The prognosis from my doctors is still vague, but I'll take the vagueness any day of the week. I think my job is to fight the vagueness with optimism.

There are a couple lessons here, the primary one being, "Don't rely on a Google search for answers to complex medical issues." But in a larger sense, the whole incident speaks to how we can deal with a prognosis that spells our mortality out in stark terms. Accurate or not, "three-and-a-half years" was a wake up call for me.

"If I heard that," said a friend of mine, "I'd curl up in a little ball and never get out of bed."

Needless to say, I didn't move in that direction. If it ever came to that, I doubt if my friend would do what he said he'd do, either. Sure, some people fall apart. But most of us put one foot in front of the other and proceed with our lives even in the face of difficult news.

We are all mortal, and in that sense every human being shares the same prognosis. It's a fact that we choose to deny or ignore as best we can. But everybody's own personal "three-and-a-half years" exists out there on the web. Once you enter in your age and other particulars, such as your health history, there are sites that will helpfully provide you with the number of years you have left to live.

If we ever find ourselves face to face with the facts, what do we do? How do we respond? I can only give insight based on my own prognosis. How long did I have to live? How long before my tumor will "light up" again or grow? More importantly, what do I do with that knowledge once I have the prognosis?

My answer to that question developed only after a period of reflection. As I've mentioned, I've always been a "real life" focused guy. I was never really into hypotheticals, and a prognosis is by definition hypothetical. It's a guess. The medical experts operate on a much higher plane than your neighborhood psychic, but the truth is that no one can know the future with any degree of certainty. I could end up surviving well beyond my doctor's predictions. Or I could step off a curb and get hit by a bus tomorrow.

So I centered in on real-life answers to the hypothetical question. I concentrated on ways to extend my life. I looked for methods to eliminate stress in my life. I began to go through ordinary day-to-day processes methodically, never wasting steps, attempting to put some order into my existence the best I could.

These measures represent my own efforts at mindfulness. From the outside, the new regimens might appear a bit anal retentive in nature, but they were simply my effort to control what I could in life. My newly developed behavioral routines were part of a natural, organic response to my prognosis. A lot of these new measures were simple common sense. I focused on healthy habits, eating right, eliminating toxins from my immediate environment, sleeping well, and resting my brain.

No more cheese dogs at midnight—in fact, I haven't had a hot dog in five years. I check out the ingredients before I even choose a facial moisturizer. The jury is still out on sunscreen because I know it is chock-full of chemicals that my pores might absorb. I exercise every day and have dropped weight. I do deep breathing exercises and meditation from time to time.

In short, I want to control what I can and avoid complex situations or problems. Not surprisingly, I've found that control, consistency, and order reduce my stress. Oddly enough, I feel healthier now than I did before my first brain surgery. It's not lost on me that though I try to avoid complex situations, I'm now pursuing the most complex of problems, the fight against cancer. Perhaps any stress associated with that effort is outweighed by the value of the cause.

I suppose a deadline helps me think and work more efficiently.

I center on actions and ideas that are meaningful. I try to get my children to think the same way, though it's an uphill battle. They don't feel the same sense of necessity that I do. Children and young adults feel immortal. For example, I've found that the pandemic doesn't frighten kids because it really doesn't impact them—until they spread the disease to a loved one. The "no fear" attitude helps explain why kids gamely set off to war when they're as young as eighteen.

The final result of all these ruminations is that I've settled on a prognosis of my own. I find myself half-jokingly saying, "I have three months or thirty years." My mindset is that I'm going for the thirty-year option. I have much more to live for. Do I still have unknowns in my life? Yes. I suppose we all do. I fight uncertainty with optimism, and I have gratitude for all the blessings I've received.

It's a good idea to stop every once in a while and ask ourselves basic questions. What's important in life? How can I live in an optimal way? What's meaningful to me? One simple question can help lead you to those others.

Tell me, what's your prognosis? Perhaps more importantly, what meaningful things are you going to do with the rest of your life?

5. Don't Expect Easy Answers to Complex Health Issues

Common sense principles involving medical issues should kick in long before a crisis hits. They may sound obvious, but they work. Some basic rules of thumb apply no matter your state of health. Stay healthy, eat right, exercise, and get good quality sleep. In general, take care of yourself. If your illness is mild, have confidence in your body's ability to beat it. Don't feel like you always have to seek medical attention.

These tried and true measures have the clear advantage of helping you to avoid a medical crisis to begin with. But even when you are faced with more serious health issues, these principles apply. Don't medicate if you don't need to. Time heals many illnesses.

My father was a doctor, and of course he was my first line of defense for medical issues that arose during my childhood. I recall accidentally cutting my arm in my youth, and the sight of the blood scared me.

What did Dad do? "Let me take a look," he said. Soberly examining the cut, he shook his head in mock seriousness. "Oh, very bad."

He was being gently sarcastic. After a few years of this same reaction, I got the message. Don't overreact. Rely on the power of the body to heal itself. If the situation is not extreme, then resist the urge to take a trip to the ER or to call 911.

I remember that my father's restrained response used to infuriate me. Didn't he care? This is the kind of treatment I get? What if my arm gets infected?

Oh, very bad.

I thought that I was the classic case of the cobbler's son getting the worst shoes. But two weeks later the cut was indeed healed and the problem had solved itself. I had already forgotten the blood, the hurt, and my dad's phlegmatic reaction. What I read as indifference was in fact my father's true wisdom.

I've noticed a similar naïve faith in medicine with my own children. Kids think medicine is an all-powerful force for healing. We have largely gotten rid of witch doctors and faith healers in favor of a scientific approach to medicine, but maybe deep-seated wishes remain. Like children, we yearn for a magic kiss-it-and-make-it-better response, a miracle potion, or a powerful, wand-waving figure that can restore us instantly to health. This leads us to seek medical care too readily, in a sort of knee-jerk response to the smallest of problems.

But when we do face a real, urgent, and serious health crisis, then we do need to seek the care of physicians. Then it becomes clear that there are few miracle cures. I recall that when I recovered from severe complications after my first brain surgery, I was really hoping it could be as simple as a magic formula to make the pain go away.

But for any serious condition, magic doesn't come into play in medicine. There is only science, and at times science can be maddeningly inexact, vague, and contradictory. I wanted clear and definite answers. But in a realm as complex as the human brain, clarity is elusive and definitive statements are rare. My recognition of this was the first step in negotiating the very real obstacles to my recovery.

My cerebellum bleed after my first craniotomy was a rare occurrence, and rarer still was the fact that the brain bleed was on the exact opposite side of the head from where my surgery occurred. With complex medical issues, don't expect perfect, rational, or consistent results.

There were other lessons that became clearer. I've learned that I have to be a determined advocate in terms of my own health care. In the first days of my medical crisis, Kim was always the point person—necessarily, because I was essentially off the planet for over two months. I wasn't even *compos mentis* enough to realize that Kim had someone stay at the home for a week after I returned from NRH.

Before my second brain surgery in early 2019, and because of the bleed I had suffered after the first surgery, we went back to check in with my hematologist. In 2018 we had learned of a 2015 letter from my hematologist to Hopkins which had discussed my condition before my first surgery. We had never seen the letter so we never had the opportunity to explore the ramifications of its contents with my medical team. That was unfortunate.

In any medical process, the first line of defense has to be the patients themselves. My wife was incredible at insisting on transparency and responsiveness during the whole ordeal. I used to hesitate when speaking with doctors. Maybe I didn't want to be rude, or perhaps I didn't want to display my ignorance. Now it's clear with all that occurred that there is no such thing as a dumb question.

I had to remind myself that doctors are just human beings too, and usually people with a lot on their plate. I was never strident or out-of-line, and I never got angry, but I wouldn't be put off, either. Kim and I learned, albeit a little too late, that we needed to insist on seeing every report, every lab result, and every single note that was being written about my case. Reading through medical documentation is frequently difficult, but it still helped us to probe further and ask the right questions.

A medical crisis is not the time to be passive. Will asking constant questions be annoying? I don't think so, but better to be annoying when your life is at stake. Plus I always found that taking an active role in understanding developments in my case helped with my mood. It was easier to remain positive when I couldn't find fault with myself for not doing enough.

Just as our physicians are not omniscient, drugs are not magical panaceas, either. I learned that I needed to extend my skeptical attitude to whatever pill was prescribed for me. The impact of drugs can be uncertain and frequently problematic, and this is especially true for their use in the long term. There is no ultimate certainty in the effect of this or that specific medicine. Sometimes steroids have a positive impact, but sometimes the side effects can be troubling. Again, as with interacting with a medical team, monitoring treatment and questioning results is not just useful, but necessary. Health advocacy doesn't stop at the pharmacy door.

Medical care is among the most complex of human disciplines. I never expect everything to go perfectly, but it's clear now that I'll always have a much better chance at medical success if I am prepared, informed, and active.

From the moment we're born, we all have the seeds of mortality sowed within us. We know it will happen, but we have no idea of the time and place of our demise or the likely cause of it.

But mostly we all just avoid giving our mortality careful regard. To the contrary, we proceed as if we might live forever. At some point the seeds of our mortality may grow. A disease may be attacking us, and we go through life without even knowing it. It can take some unexpected event to bring the truth to light. In my case, a random fender bender led to the discovery of an asymptomatic, but very serious disease.

On a scale of one to ten, how would you rate yourself as an advocate for your own state of health?

6. Finding Your Passion

We've all heard it over and over, repeated by life coaches and self-help gurus: Find your passion. These three words are easily said or recommended. And while it's definitely good advice, it's frequently difficult to achieve. I know that I risk sounding like a cliché articulating such an obvious truth, but it is a reality that has been so important to me, both during my medical crisis and throughout my life. So it drives me to emphasize it. Sure, "find your passion" is a frequently heard phrase, but that doesn't mean it's not true. And it doesn't mean it can't help someone who embraces it as a fundamental principle.

A friend of mine articulates the idea in a slightly different way: "Everyone thinks the world runs on money, but it doesn't. It runs on passion." I don't know if that's entirely true, but I remember the comedian Chris Rock offering a piece of wry wisdom. "If you have a career," he said, "don't boast about it in front of a person who just has a job." His comment gets at the difference between working for money and working because you love what you do.

I've always told my children that the perfect world is where you can combine both doing what you love and making a good living. Said another way, there is nothing better than finding a passion that pays.

In my own case, as a young man, I didn't exactly hunt down my passion like a trophy kill. Rather, I sort of fell into it. I went to law school as a fairly random choice. *Gotta do something,* I thought. I just wasn't ready to jump into the working world.

Without even realizing the value of passionate commitment, I was fortunate to have followed my passion by pursuing a career in law. The legal world has a lot of competitive aspects to it. Generating business, crafting the most effective argument, appearing in front of a mediator or an arbitration panel—these were activities during my law career in which I thrived. I was good at them because I had a passion for competing and prevailing. I also felt I had good common sense, which I found to be very helpful in practicing law and handling cases.

Here's another way to find your passion. Base your search on your direct experience. I grew up participating in sports, especially becoming deeply involved in wrestling. I honed my competitive spirit. I came to learn what motivated me.

I recall losing to an opponent during our first match, but then beating him in our next two matches. Once an opponent has beaten you, it's very difficult mentally to then turn around and beat him. When I won those subsequent two matches, I felt like I was on top of the world. Memories about key events in life don't fade. Those wins have stayed indelibly etched in my mind for over forty-five years.

If you discover your passion within your own experience, then it is not some abstract concept, but a living, breathing reality. Again and again, I've returned to the mindset of wrestling for inspiration in achieving difficult goals in life.

My son Garrett, also a wrestler, knows by heart a line that we exchange once in a while when the going gets tough. It emerged out of a difficult match during Garrett's own long wrestling career, where he came from behind and prevailed in the last thirty seconds of the match.

"Down by two, thirty seconds left—gut it out."

That's become a favorite line with Garrett and me. It speaks to the energy and motivation that can be derived from accomplishing something you are passionate about.

Finding your passion and making a living following your passion is not easy. Such a gift won't just drop out of the sky. At times in my own life, I've had to just sit down and give it some good hard thought. For me, it took feeling the pleasure of a hard-fought match to see that I was passionate about competing. And it wasn't really about wrestling per se; it was the satisfaction I felt after working hard, competing, and winning.

What makes it hard for people to discover their true passion? Fear of failure might be involved. Or an uncertain frame of mind. Maybe the best thing for many of us to do is to see a career advisor with whom you can explore your potential career passion in a meaningful way. I never pursued this career consulting approach, but in retrospect, I should have.

The wife of a friend endured two years of cooking school, which involved a lot of arduous labor in a hot kitchen, much of it scutwork. Ultimately she wanted to become a chef. She went through the whole program, graduated, and then decided she really didn't want to do restaurant work after all. I suppose the path to becoming a chef just wasn't her passion.

Another friend of mine is someone who is a very capable guy, presentable, personable, and well-spoken. He can do a lot of great things and has a lot of talent, but finding true success has been a bit elusive for him. He appreciated this issue and described his work ethic to me: "Tell me what you want me to do—I'll do it and I'll do it well."

He was stuck a couple of levels below leadership in his company. I felt he could easily take on a top management role. He might even enjoy it and, in that way, it could help him see his passion. A life that isn't self-directed is still worth living, but it lacks getting to the heart of what one really wants to do and should be doing.

As I said, because of my medical crisis I've found a new passion, which is to help in the fight against cancer. It's definitely an important endeavor, and it gets me up in the morning in a positive frame of mind. I have a goal, and the goal is meaningful, interesting, and important. Finding your passion may actually lead to a longer life, precisely because you will feel you have an important mission to accomplish.

Finding passion in your work is the ideal. Perhaps it's working on a medical breakthrough or maybe it's developing a cutting-edge communication process to connect "smart cities" throughout the world. Whatever it may be, finding work that you love is locating the true sweet spot in life.

Having a mission helps you to power ahead with your work. It's the fuel of existence. Never overlook the fact that happiness is found in leading a life based on passion, character, integrity, and honesty, as well as knowing that those around you love and appreciate you. The struggles you will encounter along the way are troubling, but I believe they're intended to shape your purpose.

Are you pursuing your passion in life?

7 . Turn Perceived Weaknesses into Strengths (And Don't Be Deceived by Appearances)

In the aftermath of my medical crisis, I find myself getting mis-judged all the time. By that I mean some people assume I'm stronger than I am and that I have more energy than I really do. Why do people think that way? I think it's understandable. While I look reasonably healthy and fit, in truth I more resemble that bad cell phone you had that needed frequent recharging.

"Ten a.m. tee-time," announced a friend of mine on the phone. He was an old golf buddy from way back, and we had talked about getting out on the links.

"I don't think that works for me," I told him.

"What do you mean?" my friend said.

"I definitely can't manage a full round of golf."

"What's the issue?" he inquired further. He just wasn't getting it. I had to lay it all out for him. I told him that I no longer had the endurance to make more than nine holes.

"But you're recovered, aren't you? You look fine!" I thought to myself, *are you kidding?* I had survived a near-death experience.

"They almost laid me out on a slab!"

Frankly, I'm glad that I can still play golf, despite an impact to the vision in my left eye due to a radiation side effect. I'm not ready for the pro tour, but I still get out there and hit 'em from time to time.

I may look good physically. I might even appear healthier

than I did pre-surgery. But physically and mentally, I just cannot do the same things I did without a problem. I tire out quickly. I avoid complex facts, lengthy reading, and writing exercises, or speech and speech projection efforts. Speech projection is very tiring and just wipes me out. Despite a lot of help, the drafting of this book has taken me over six years. I'm forced to nap a lot. But none of my impediments would be obvious from just a casual glance at me walking down the street.

There are a couple conclusions I can draw from this situation. Don't judge anyone by their appearance, because appearances are often deceiving. In fact, maybe hold off judging other people altogether. Better heed the advice often attributed to the philosopher Plato: "Be kind, because everyone you meet is carrying a heavy burden."

Another takeaway is that if you find yourself in my situation, if you have developed a new vulnerability or find your old ways beyond your reach, don't despair. Instead, try to discover a new path, one that turns your weaknesses into strength. Yes, of course, always capitalize on your strengths, but also seize the opportunity to develop your weaknesses into further strengths.

These days I don't have the stamina or focus for the challenges of the long and arduous hours of my legal practice. I'm not the same guy I once was, but I'm still me. Sure my horsepower is way down, but I'm hoping my values have become more focused and positive. My personality might have changed for the better since I'm unfettered by work demands. My mind is generally intact, and that's saying something for a guy who's had part of his brain removed. I always try to judge how my illness has impacted me, and make adjustments in order to do the things I want to do.

It's as if I've been traded to a new team, or like I've been drafted by God to do a different kind of work. I can imagine the universe shifting under my feet. The Fates spoke. *Oh, that guy, the one who is spending all his talents and energy on legal cases, well, we're going to transfer him to another, more important job.* Maybe someone thought that slugging it out in legal disputes was not the best use of my time. *We cannot have him do this law stuff, that's too narrow of a focus. Helping in the fight against cancer,* whispered the gods, *that's the life for him.*

I don't want people thinking, oh, poor Bob. The enormous changes I've experienced in my life are not of my choice, but I can clearly see the positive side. I am putting my energy into the effort to help find a cure for cancer. It's something of a calling, an important mission in life, an opportunity to help out in the world in a more meaningful way. In short, I've chosen to take my weaknesses and do something productive with them.

Turn your weaknesses into your strengths. I always tell my kids not to give too much thought to their own appearance or how they come off to others. "Don't worry about what people think of you. They're probably too worried about what you think about them."

We are all mostly locked within our own bubbles, and I think that's even truer the younger you are. Many under twenty-five are fighting political and other causes. But still many are living in the age of the selfie. They expend a lot of energy trying to look perfect on Instagram. It almost seems that the younger set looks to go on vacations just for the perfect selfie to send to their friends, posed in front of the Pyramids, the Eiffel Tower, or the Great Wall of China.

Even in my diminished state, I try to bring what I can to the table. So I can't handle billion-dollar law suits anymore. I still find that I can apply some of the skills I developed in my career as a lawyer to my new mission of fundraising for the cancer fight. For example, from practicing law I learned how to cut through distractions and get to the heart of a problem. I can still marshal the greatest resource of them all, human energy, by networking among friends, associates, and experts. That's what I did in my professional life, and that's what I can still do now.

Don't judge me by my appearance, for either better or for worse. I may seem strong, but cancer has weakened me in ways that might not be readily apparent. On the other hand, my medical crisis has had the positive impact of forcing me to develop important new strengths, paths, and goals.

How have you been misjudged in your own life? How can you capitalize on both your strengths and weaknesses to make a real difference in the world?

8. Seeing the Significance in the Seemingly Insignificant

Life ultimately becomes a game of connect the dots. This happened, which then triggered something else to happen, and on and on, past to present, from birth to where we are today. It can be a diverting game to trace the connections and to consider how we arrived at our current circumstance.

I've had a lot of time to think about the chain of events that have led me to my present circumstances. What's clear to me is that significant developments don't always announce themselves at the time. We see them for what they are only in retrospect. This has led me to a further conclusion that I should look for significance even in the seemingly insignificant.

Meeting Mitchel Berger, the doctor who performed the second surgery on my brain tumor, qualifies as a momentous development in my life. Dr. Berger is one of the finest neurosurgeons in the world. As a professor and chair of Neurological Surgery at the University of California, San Francisco, he works at a very high level. Just to give one example among the many technical matters he focuses on, he was a co-principal investigator on a research study entitled "Noninvasive Metabolic Signatures to Improve Management of Molecular Subtypes of Glioma," funded by the National Institutes of Health's National Cancer Institute.

But Dr. Berger is based in San Francisco, while I live in the

Washington, DC area. How were those two particular dots connected?

Several months after my first surgery, when I was still in recovery from the catastrophic brain bleed that almost killed me, I found myself at the Dabbiere's home for the "Grey Soiree," a cancer fundraising event.

I recall thinking at the event, how could a gathering of so many cancer survivors take place on an uneven side lawn? Didn't anyone understand how difficult it was for someone in my condition to walk across a lawn? Smooth-polished floors and flat surfaces only, please. About a month or so after the soiree, it dawned on me that I was probably the only one fresh off the debilitating effects of a stroke. So on reflection, the location of the event now made total sense.

Kim chose not to attend the Grey Soiree. She was feeling a little overwhelmed by the relatively recent focus on cancer in our lives. I understood how it could be a bit much for her. Cancer research, cancer fundraising, cancer recovery. I went through my medical treatment literally comatose and pretty much oblivious, while Kim was forced to watch it all unfold in real time.

I didn't stay long at the Grey Soiree. Fortunately, I did have a brief meet-and-greet with Ashley Dabbiere, and we agreed to get together for lunch to talk about all we had both been through.

A cascade of connections and events followed. At the time, I hardly realized the significance of meeting Ashley. I was barely in shape to realize the significance of anything. But many months down the road, Ashley Dabbiere would introduce me to Dr. Mitchel Berger. She had interviewed a lot of doctors before she settled on him for her surgery. She described Berger as more or less God's gift to dealing with my kind of tumor. When my brain cancer recurred, it was Dr. Berger who urged immediate surgical intervention, instead of a course of radiation and chemotherapy that other doctors counseled.

Looking back, I can play the game of "what if?" What if Kim had never reached out to Brock Green? What if Ashley Dabbiere lived in Houston or Chicago, instead of right next door in McLean, Virginia? I would have never gone to the Grey Soiree. It's true that I might have connected up with Dr. Berger via another route. But I might not have.

Connect the dots: a fender bender to an MRI to brain surgery to a devastating stroke; Kim's proactive approach, leading to Brock Green, who led me to Ashley Dabbiere, who in turn led me to Dr. Berger.

Miracles can seem to crop up at random, almost by mistake. A brain tumor might have been God's way of getting me to focus on a more important challenge. It's awful to think so, and at the same time it's awesome to think so, too.

My medical crisis helped me to understand that significance can be hidden within insignificant occurrences. Miracles happen, and their occurrence is not always immediately obvious. The miracles may be very small. On the other hand, miracles may be quite significant.

As it turns out, I've had the benefit of plenty of miracles associated with my medical experience, but it took me some reflection to realize that they were truly miracles. I have learned to adopt a much lower standard when I rate this or that event in terms of significance. Too many minor things have happened to me that have turned out to have major repercussions.

I have never wanted to put too much weight on my own importance. What's significant for me won't be the same as it is for you. All I'm suggesting is that there can be meaning and importance in the smallest happening—"a universe in a grain of sand," as the poet William Blake put it.

In a very real sense, a lot of the life I led has become more insignificant since my medical crisis. I have been sidelined from the law. Stick me in the middle of a law case today, and I could not perform. The details, multiple variables, and constant back and forth in a complicated legal proceeding would wipe me out both mentally and physically. As for the hours of concentrated study required to handle a legal matter, forget it.

I recently walked our neighborhood with Kim and a representative from our local homeowner's association. After only a few minutes, the fire hose of information coming at me forced me to leave, go home, and take a nap.

I see that I'm finding more meaning and significance in what most others would just view as the day-to-day. For example, in the summer after my first brain surgery, I recall when three generations of the Brams men went to a baseball game: Dad, Garrett, and I. Dad's beloved Philadelphia Phillies beat the Washington Nationals' ace pitcher, Max Scherzer. While it should have been terribly hot and humid, the weather in DC on this August afternoon was absolutely perfect.

Dad, now ninety-two, could not have been more thrilled with the outing, and he told me that he appreciated that this might be the last game he would attend in person. Nevertheless, his tone and attitude were still quite positive. We all left the game in good spirits. While it was just a simple baseball game, for me that day had plenty of significance.

The lesson here is to participate in enjoyable and meaningful experiences in life and appreciate the happiness they bring. Of course, every day we wake up alive is a miracle of sorts, an event of truly shattering significance. Yet I used to accept it as just another day. A brush with mortality taught me much differently.

Where do you find significance in your life?

9. Live Without Fear

I call it the "hit by a bus" factor. For some reason, that's a common reference point when people consider the randomness of fate. As in, "Today I could quit smoking, quit drinking, and stop eating fast food, then step off a curb tomorrow and get hit by a bus." I've checked up on this, and of course people do indeed die by being hit by buses. There were thirty-three such fatalities in 2017, the last year for which I could find statistics.

The whole idea of randomness speaks to the "known" and the "unknown" elements in life. There will always be the "hit by a bus" unknown, developments too random to be predicted. This could involve rampaging public transportation, or it could be a meteor. The unknown is always worrisome, but it is usually too remote to be seriously considered.

On the other hand, there are the known factors in our mortality. In my case, the known factor is brain cancer. Yes, a brain tumor may kill me. It's my known quantity, and I'll fight the cancer battle hard. But I really don't know what might kill me, since people don't really know what may take them down.

A known mortality factor is both a curse and, oddly enough, a blessing. I can look up statistics to determine brain cancer survival rates. As I've said previously, early on during my medical crisis, I did this and it sobered the hell out of me. But it also focused my priorities, so in that respect, my possible death sentence was a blessing.

The reaction to human mortality is basic, fundamental, and almost universal. *We don't want to know.* We're destined to die from the day we're born, but we don't lead our lives paralyzed by that fear. In fact, we customarily talk about the day of our deaths as if today is not the day. "We know not the day or the hour," as the Bible states it. With the pandemic that 2020 unleashed upon the world, people were faced with the fact of their own mortality in concrete and ever-present ways, most probably for the first time.

I've had six years to think about that serious risk. My conclusion is a truth that most everyone seems to put forth, from the great philosophers to Hallmark greeting card writers.

Live every day as if it might be your last.

In the various combat theaters of the Middle East, this principle comes up again and again in interviews of people in war-torn areas. When your life is always in danger, you simply try to make the best of your day-to-day existence. Survivors of the civil war in Syria, for example, live with the fact of their mortality staring them in the face. In Israel, the threat is not so immediate, but ever-present nonetheless. From afar I detect a certain life-affirming joy on the part of Israeli citizens. It's as if the constant possibility of attack has not robbed them of their ability to enjoy themselves, but rather has rendered them more determined to wring every bit of life out of their existence.

In societies not under threat of immediate attack, living every day like it might be your last sounds a bit extreme. The point is to live responsibly, but never in fear. The truth is that we all exist under a death sentence. We might not like it, we might avoid thinking about it, and we might deny it to our last breath. I am living testimony that the alternative is not only possible, but can be unexpectedly rewarding.

One crucial step I took in response to my medical crisis was to put my affairs in order. We all generally feel some relief from stress when we get organized and clear clutter from our lives. I've already planned my estate, written my will, and formulated directives for how I want my death handled. Attending to these matters took a weight off my shoulders.

Writing up my wishes in legalese was helpful, but it really didn't address every detail of ensuring my family was well prepared to successfully proceed through life in the event of my death. Fortunately my kids have college degrees. What paths do they have in mind for successful careers? What level of financial support would they need to get them through difficult times? I can't tie up every loose end, but I have done what I can to ensure that my children are able to rationally think through problems on their own that may arise in their own lives.

Many of us avoid putting our affairs in order because it means facing up to the fact of our eventual passing. The statistics say 60 percent of Americans have not prepared wills or estate planning. I definitely see the whole estate planning process as staring into the face of my demise, but the upside is so real and deep that any discomfort is worth it. But even greater comfort comes when you feel your spouse and your children are on reasonably solid economic footing. Will my children be secure when it comes to their educations, careers, relationships, and overall safety and health? Nothing is certain, but I believe my children are heading in the right direction.

As I write this, the sad news comes of the passing of *Jeopardy!* host Alex Trebek. I admired and agreed with many of the statements he made about his mortality while he was still with us. "One thing they're not going to say at my funeral during a eulogy is 'he was taken from us too soon,'" he said. "I'm seventy-nine years old. I've lived a full life, a good life, and I'm nearing the end of that life. I know that. I'm not going to delude myself. If it happens, it happens. Why should I be afraid of that?"

However, I'm not eighty years old, I'm *only* sixty-one years old—just a spring chicken. There's more I want to see and do in life, like attending the weddings of my children, becoming grandparents together with Kim, and seeing my family's further achievements. I must confess that I'd like another thirty years or so. Is that asking too much? I don't think so!

What are your thoughts and strategies concerning your own mortality? What are you really looking forward to?

10. Gather Knowledge and Inspire the Next Generation

Supporting our families, properly raising our children, and helping others may be our most important jobs in life. For me, that means putting kids out in the world with character, integrity, and with the intelligence and desire to have a positive impact on others. Stated simply, everyone's goal should be to strive to become a good person.

The idea of passing down knowledge has been brought home to me more and more due to my brush with mortality. When you're knocking at death's door, a lot of things become crystal clear. I thought of how my parents raised me, how their parents raised them, and on and on in a long chain that stretches into the distant past. Patterns of behavior are passed on just like your grandfather's gold heirloom watch.

You can't do everything for your kids. You can tell them about the lessons you've learned, but unless and until they've gone through experiences themselves, they might still need to test things. Trying to live their lives for them interferes with one of our main objectives, which should be inculcating a spirit of independence. Unless you can manage to raise creative and independent thinkers, your failure will become apparent when you pass away and you aren't around to support and nurture them.

During my recovery after my first surgery, when I had death

staring me in the face, my thoughts returned again and again to the very basic question of the best way to raise my children. How do you get your kids to listen to you? How can you best prepare them to overcome the obstacles that will surface in their lives?

One thing I decided was that any truth I had to impart had to come from my own experience. I could read all the parenting books in the world, but my own life provided the best lessons.

Out of this thought came the conviction that at times the road less traveled could be the best path to take. In my life I did not follow the best, most widely accepted path to success. Early on, I failed to focus properly on academics. Then I went from one law school to another. So is this the model I want to impart to my children?

Not really. I guess the lesson is that if you can hit all the marks on the path more regularly traveled, if you can succeed academically and attend the finest schools and make the best contacts, by all means, go that more standard route. But if for whatever reason that well-traveled path is not available to you, or somehow it's just not working for you, don't despair. It may be the time to choose the road less traveled, to embrace it and take pleasure in it.

I don't normally like to see the kind of over-parenting that is all too common nowadays. The DC area, where I live, is the home of many ferocious high-achievers, who watch over their children like hawks. I find this style of parenting to be overbearing. But I've come to think that some degree of "helicoptering" is absolutely necessary in today's cultural environment. The world has become a much more complicated place.

I was raised in such a way that my mom and dad could watch me slam out the back door of the house, jump on my bike, and disappear for a whole afternoon without knowing precisely what I was up to. That sort of freedom was priceless in shaping my character. But it was a very different world back then. Nowadays who knows what's lurking in the streets? What dangers infest social media? I monitor my children more closely than my parents did back in the day.

One of the roles I've taken seriously as a parent is trying to give my kids an understanding of the financial realities of life. If they are on a path to a career where they'll start off making fifteen dollars an hour in New York City, for example, I want them to realize they won't be able to afford high-end clothing or restaurant meals, and they won't be able to pay rent on even a small apartment unless they have roommates.

Of course, it's not where you start, but rather where you finish. So a fifteen-dollar-an-hour internship might be the best move at an early stage in one's career. My own legal internship and clerkship turned out to be crucial in shaping my professional life. But all students need to look ahead and see what awaits them. They need to realize what it takes to make monthly payments on a car, to buy a house, or to send their own children to college. Beyond all this, there's the often overlooked necessity of saving money. Life is not as easy or simple as it may appear to the young adult mind.

We all live in a world where every day seems to have more distractions than the day before. I witness my children trying to manage to have a dinner table conversation while at the same time attending to text messages on their phones. Kim and I try to enforce a rule of no cell phone usage at the dinner table.

We've arrived at a point where multitasking is a virtue. I've heard Bill Gates suggest that we might be confusing being busy with being successful. I remember a video presentation where Gates displayed the activity calendar of his friend Warren Buffett. It featured just three entries for almost every week.

What could one of the most successful investors of all time possibly be doing with all that blank space in his days? The point Bill Gates made, one with which Warren Buffett readily agreed, is that Buffett found his time was frequently best spent just thinking. I'm sure some of that time was taken up by trying to determine what he was passionate about pursuing. Buffett's overriding passion was finding smart business deals and investing. He just didn't want to get caught up in doing busy-work that had no potential.

Buffett had developed tremendous insight for seeing which businesses would likely be most successful. It struck me that his professional life had almost become like a game to him. He lived a very modest lifestyle, treating himself to some fine dining almost every morning at McDonalds. After spending a couple of bucks for breakfast, he would then head off to work a make a billion dollars on deals. Nice work if you can get it! I still believe some brainstorming sessions with other intelligent people can have real value. I suspect Buffett would probably agree

So these are a few of the lessons I've tried to pass on to my children. Consider the road less traveled. Allow for some helicopter parenting. Don't confuse being busy as a sign of success. Because those conclusions arose from my personal experience, they tend toward what today is termed a "normative" frame of mind But I believe that even if one does not live in a two-parent household with one-point-nine-three children, it's still possible to model behaviors that will have a positive impact on others.

What are you interested in passing on to the next generation?

11. Being Right Doesn't Always Mean You Should Push Your Position

Just because you're the one in the right in a disagreement, don't expect to arrive at a solution that proves your point. Sometimes you can take a position that you know is totally correct, that you can prove rationally, but it's still not worth the repercussions of an argument.

A better option might be getting to a compromise solution with which you can live, one that seems fair and reasonable. You avoid the stress, mental anguish, and cost of proving yourself right. A fast and fair resolution can actually be a less taxing outcome. Consciously aim to decide a matter quickly, even if the solution is not perfect or not what it should be. Move on to greener pastures and calmer waters. Perhaps afterward you can consider how to avoid the same kind of dispute in the future.

Arguments, debates, and court battles are messy. They can take a lot out of you. There's an old expression, "The game isn't worth the candle." It's about a card game that is such a losing proposition, or so unexciting, uncompetitive, or downright boring, that it's not worth burning a candle to play the game.

Likewise, before entering a dispute, it's a good idea to ask yourself if it's worth your while to bother.

Part of this is purely about stress reduction. Hypothetically, I'm in a position where I know I've been harmed by another person's actions. I know I'm right, and I could even go to court and prove it.

What do I do? Do I rush off to court? Or do I stop and just think, pause, and reflect on how I should proceed? A legal battle can take months, even years. The expense in terms of time and money can be significant, and the process can weigh heavily on your mind. Pursuing court suits brings on stress.

In addition, an argument or lawsuit often results in burned bridges. Do I really want to alienate another person, especially one with whom I might need to work in the future? One must think carefully about the consequences involved.

For me, given my condition, there are simple questions I ask myself before raising an issue in personal matters. Did the person act intentionally or out of malice? Or was the person acting in earnest and in good faith? This may be a good standard to follow before even raising an issue. Everyone makes mistakes. Consider rising above the fray. Money is not everything. Being right is not everything. Sometimes the better way is for all parties to forgive and move on.

What exactly are we seeking by raising something to the level of a dispute? Is it the damage or loss we've suffered? Is it to be "made whole" by the judgment awarded by a court? This idea doesn't take into account the hassle, worry, and bridges burned involved in getting to a solution that favors us. Maybe the matter involves a fundamental issue that needs to be asserted to make an important point. Disputes take on many shapes and sizes. The answer is sometimes elusive.

Beyond financial relief, maybe we seek something deeper, more intangible. We want validation. We want the court—which stands for the world in general—to tell us we are right. We want a third party to tell our adversary that they're wrong.

I've spent a great deal of my life involved in legal matters, so I'm framing the question in terms of lawsuits and court judgments. But the same principles apply in our day-to-day lives. Disputes occasionally arise within the family or among friends.

In the aftermath of my medical crisis, and in my life with family members, friends, and acquaintances, I've changed the way I approach arguments and disputes. I check myself and rein in my urge to be right. In the grand scheme of things, being right turns out not to matter at all.

This is especially true with those I hold near and dear. All the members of my immediate family are strong-minded. The question might be minor, but everyone has an opinion on it. Lately I've tried to be more flexible and to give way much more. Does it really matter? How often do I argue just to argue, trying to attain that ever-elusive validation?

A small example: My wife and I were looking to install a new shower head. If you've walked down the plumbing aisle lately, you know there are almost a comical number of choices. I had my own opinion and I knew Kim had hers, too. Do I indulge in a debate over how forceful the water should come out of the shower head jets? I don't think so. Not important at all.

There are countless issues that arise around the home. The color of paint for a kitchen remodeling, the style of lighting above the stove—what is really so important about all these day-to-day decisions? Why should I allow them to cause me angst? In my former life I might have put up more of an argument over the color of paint or the choice of a shower head, but in my present frame of mind those issues are very small and inconsequential. I just walk away without giving much thought to voicing my preferences. The result just doesn't matter.

I've learned the value of choosing my battles. When I think about disagreements that may arise in my life these days, I've come to realize that a lot of them are easily dismissed as simply "not worth the candle." I've chosen to fight one big battle—the battle against cancer—and that has put all other battles in perspective. THIS is actually an important issue.

What do you think is worth fighting for?

12. Finding Value in Writing About Your Experience

Have you ever noticed that pretty much all the advice other people dole out can be distilled down to three words? "Be like me."

I've tried to offer insights and wisdom that came to me only after living through a near-death experience. Many of these ideas became clearer to me only after I tried to write them down. So I want to suggest a similar course of action for anyone seeking to determine their own values, their own wisdom, and their own essence. I almost hesitate to suggest it, but "be like me." Write down your thoughts and feelings. Tell your own story.

I find writing to be therapeutic and cathartic. Some prefer talk therapy. Both approaches involve the use of language to clarify what might otherwise be vague concepts and inchoate experiences. We might think we know the ideas that fuel our thoughts, but writing them down brings them into sharper focus. Even if it goes no further than a drawer in your desk, it can be a bracing exercise.

There's another value involved here. Writing or journaling can have incredible significance for your family and others down the road. Your writing will take its place as a part of your family history. If expressing your thoughts through writing them down can lead to greater clarity in your own thinking, it could possibly lead to greater clarity in your family's thinking, too.

Socrates, a philosopher famed for wisdom, but who modestly labeled himself the most ignorant man in Athens, formulated a famous precept at the end of his life: "The unexamined life is not worth living," he said. Writing down an account of your experiences, your beliefs, and your accumulated wisdom can be the best way to lead an examined life, a life worth living.

What's the first sentence of your written account of your own life?

Always Remember, It's Not Where You Start, It's Where You Finish.

Acknowledgments

First and foremost, I'd like to express gratitude to my family—my father, my mother (Mom passed away on March 30, 2020, and I miss her every day), my brother, my wife. and my son and daughter—for their endless support throughout my medical crisis and during the effort involved in writing this book. I could not have done it without you and love you very much.

I would like to express my appreciation for all the invaluable help I (really my team) received from the wonderful group at Skyhorse Publishing, including Tony Lyons, Mark Gompertz, Caroline Russomanno, and Kathleen Schmidt, as well as a number of others offering key support.

I acknowledge the generosity of donors who have responded or will respond to my appeal for support in the fight against brain cancer. Donors are recognized at the website: **1MBBC.com**.

Resources

Air Charity Network
(877) 621–7177
www.aircharitynetwork.org
Air Charity Network is a charitable organization that provides access for people in need who are seeking free air transportation to specialized health care facilities or distant destinations due to family, community, or national crisis.

Alex's Lemonade Stand Foundation
(866) 333–1213
www.alexslemonade.org
Alex's Lemonade Stand Foundation (ALSF) offers help to children with cancer via many programs, including funding research, raising awareness, and supporting families.

Allyson Whitney Foundation (Young Adults)
www.allysonwhitney.org
The Foundation's vision is to shine a spotlight on an underserved demographic of young adults with cancer and to place an emphasis on the need for rare cancer research. The Foundation

primarily provides individuals with "Life Interrupted Grants" to ease their financial burden so that they can concentrate their energy on healing.

America's Pharmacy
(888) 495–3181
www.americaspharmacy.com
Prescription savings program accepted in over 62,000 pharmacies across the US.

American Brain Tumor Association (ABTA)
(800) 886–2282
www.abta.org
ABTA raises funds for brain tumor research and education; their website offers information, education, and support.

American Cancer Society (ACS)
(800) 227–2345
www.cancer.org
ACS offers information about brain tumors, treatments, and managing life with the disease; a search tool helps locate support groups; ACS offers the Health Insurance Assistance Service.

Brain Tumor Network
(844) 286–6110
www.braintumornetwork.org
Free internet navigation resource for brain tumor patients and caregivers.

Brain Tumor Copayment Assistance Program
(855) 426–2672
www.braintumorcopays.org
This program provides up to five thousand dollars in financial assistance per year to families who qualify and use certain drugs to treat brain tumors.

Cameron Siemers Foundation for Hope
www.cameronsiemers.org
Each year, the Cameron Siemers Foundation for Hope awards a minimum of four Life Grants to young adults who are living with life-threatening illnesses. A Life Grant is an award of up to five thousand dollars to help young adults make a difference in their lives and their communities.

Camp Kesem
(253) 736–3821
www.campkesem.org
Provides free summer camp for children of parents with cancer.

Cancer.net
(888) 651–3038
www.cancer.net
Cancer.net is a resource for direct and accurate information about cancer treatment based on the expertise of clinical oncologists.

Cancer and Careers (CAC)
(646) 929–8032
www.cancerandcareers.org
CAC educates people with cancer to thrive in their workplace.

Look online for free publications, career coaching, and support groups for employees with cancer.

CancerCare
(800) 813–4673
www.cancercare.org
CancerCare offers limited financial assistance for cancer-related costs such as transportation and child care, and their oncology social workers can help you find resources.

Cancer for College
(760) 599–5096
www.cancerforcollege.org
College scholarships for cancer patients.

Cancer Horizons
www.cancerhorizons.com
(801) 501–7500
Provides resources for financial support in terms of rent, housing, medical bills, caregiver assistance, life insurance funding, and legal assistance.

Cancer Legal Resource Center (CLRC)
(866) 843–2572
www.CancerLegalResourceCenter.org
The CLRC provides free and confidential information and resources on cancer-related legal issues for anyone coping with cancer.

Cancer Survivors' Fund
(281) 437–7142
www.cancersurvivorsfund.org
Cancer Survivors' Fund is a non-profit organization that provides college scholarships and prosthetics for the benefit of persons diagnosed with cancer, receiving treatment for cancer, or in remission, with the aim of giving them a new purpose and meaning in life.

Cancer Support Community (CSC)
(888) 793–9355
www.cancersupportcommunity.org
The Cancer Support Community offers a wide array of resources. CSC's Helpline is staffed by licensed counselors available to assist. Sixty locations plus more than one hundred satellites around the country offer on-site support groups, educational workshops, yoga, nutrition, and mind-body programs specifically designed for people affected by cancer.

Centers for Medicare & Medicaid Services
(800) 633–4227
www.cms.gov
A Federal program providing guidance to Medicaid, Medicare, and the Health Insurance Exchanges.

Compassion Can't Wait
(310) 276–7111
www.compassioncantwait.org
When compassion can't wait and single parent families are in

despair, this organization helps with urgent expenses to allow these caregivers to stay at their child's bedside during catastrophic illness.

Co-Pay Relief Program (CPR)
(866) 512–3861
www.copays.org
The CPR program provides financial support to insured patients who qualify to access pharmaceutical co-pay assistance. The program offers call counselors who guide patients through the enrollment process.

Corporate Angel Network
(866) 328–1313
www.corpangelnetwork.org
Corporate Angel Network is a non-profit organization that arranges free air transportation for cancer patients traveling to treatment using the empty seats on corporate jets.

FinAid
www.finaid.org/?s=cancer
Database of scholarships for cancer patients, survivors, and others touched by cancer.

First Descents
(303) 945–2490
www.firstdescents.org
Provides guided adventures for young cancer patients.

Foundation for Appropriate and Immediate Temporary Help
(FAITH) (Northern Virginia)
(571) 323–2198
www.faithus.org
Helps families in the northern areas of Virginia with immediate
and temporary support in areas of rent, mortgage, utilities, education, and medical bills.

Good Days
(877) 968–7233
www.mygooddays.org
Helps patients who have limited financial means access the
medications they need. Their program helps qualified patients
pay their insurance co-pays so they can get immediate access to
prescription medications. Their program also helps with transportation and lodging needs. Check their website for up-to-date
covered diagnoses.

GoodRX
(855) 268–2822
www.goodrx.com
Prescription discount card program. Helps identify pharmacies
providing the lowest price for your medications.

Greg's Mission
(612) 437–5903
www.gregsmission.org
Greg's Mission is a non-profit that provides support, hope, education, current resources, and awareness to patients suffering from
brain tumors, especially Glioblastoma Multiforme (a Grade IV
primary brain tumor).

The Healing Exchange (T.H.E.) Brain Trust
(877) 252–8480
www.braintrust.org
T.H.E. Brain Trust runs online support groups and forums for discussion of all brain tumors for patients, providers, researchers, educators, and caregivers.

Healthcare.gov
(800) 318–2596
www.healthcare.gov
The Federal website offering customized information about the various health insurance options for which you may be eligible, including comprehensive information about Medicare and Medicare Services through www.cms.gov.

Healthcare Hospitality Network
www.hhnetwork.org/find-lodging#/
HHN is a nationwide professional association of nearly 200 unique, non-profit organizations that provide lodging and support services to patients, families and their loved ones who are receiving medical treatment far from their home communities.

HealthWell Foundation
(800) 675–8416
www.healthwellfoundation.org
Provides financial assistance to eligible individuals to cover coinsurance, copayments, health care premiums, and deductibles for certain medications and therapies. Focus of disease funding varies, so check their website for an up-to-date list of covered diagnoses and medications.

Hope Lodge

(800) 227–2345

www.cancer.org/treatment/support-programs-and-services/
patient-lodging/hope-lodge.html

Some hospital systems have Hope Lodge, a place for caregivers
to stay during treatment and recovery. Check to see if your hospital has a Hope Lodge. Each Hope Lodge offers cancer patients
and their caregivers a free place to stay when their best hope for
effective treatment may be in another city. Hope Lodge provides
a nurturing, home-like environment where guests can retreat to
private rooms or connect with others. Every Hope Lodge also
offers a variety of resources and information about cancer and
how best to fight the disease.

Imerman Angels

(312) 274–5529

www.imermanangels.org

Imerman Angels matches anyone seeking cancer support with
someone just like you—a "Mentor Angel" who is the same age,
gender, and has beaten the same type of cancer.

Inheritance of Hope

(914) 213–8435

www.inheritanceofhope.org

Provides retreats for families who have a parent diagnosed with
a terminal illness.

Joe's House

(877) 563-7468

www.joeshouse.org

The Joe's House website lists thousands of places to stay across the country near hospitals and treatment centers that offer a discount for traveling patients and their loved ones.

LawHelp.org

www.LawHelp.org

LawHelp.org helps low and moderate income people find free legal aid programs in their communities, answers questions about legal rights, and helps with their legal problems.

Lifeline Pilots

(800) 822-7972

www.lifelinepilots.org

Facilitates free transportation for such medical needs as ongoing medical treatments, diagnosis and follow-up care.

Livestrong Foundation

(855) 220-7777

www.livestrong.org/cancersupport

The Livestrong Foundation provides information and tools to help people affected by cancer. Livestrong Navigation Services offers free referrals and other resources in your area.

Love, Team Tessa

www.loveteamtessa.org

Helps with groceries, bills, fuels, transportation costs, and medication co-pays.

Medicine Assistance Tool

www.medicineassistancetool.org

A search engine designed to help patients, caregivers, and health-care providers learn more about the resources available through the various biopharmaceutical industry programs.

Musella Foundation for Brain Tumor Research

(888) 295–4740

www.virtualtrials.com

Musella Foundation offers education, support (emotional and financial), advocacy, and guidance to brain tumor patients. Videos, articles, online support groups, and information about fundraisers for brain tumor research are also available.

National Brain Tumor Society (NBTS)

(800) 770–8287

www.braintumor.org

NBTS drives strategic research to find new treatments and advocates for policies to meet the critical needs of this community.

National Cancer Institute (NCI)

(800) 422–6237

www.cancer.gov

NCI is the premier agency for cancer research, training, and information in the US Federal Government. Their website has valuable information for all people affected by cancer—including search tools for clinical trials.

National Cancer Legal Services Network (NCLSN)
www.NCLSN.org
NCLSN is a coalition of legal service providers who offer some free legal services programs to people affected by cancer.

National Center for Comprehensive and Alternative Medicine (NCCAM)
(888) 644–6226
www.nccam.nih.gov
NCCAM is the Federal Government's lead agency for scientific research on the practices known as comprehensive and alternative medicine (CAM). NCCAM offers information on the value and legitimacy of CAM practices.

National Coalition for Cancer Survivorship (NCCS)
(888) 650–9127
www.canceradvocacy.org
NCCS offers free publications on insurance and employment issues for people coping with cancer. The Cancer Survival Toolbox is an audio program that includes a section on "Finding Ways to Pay for Care."

National Collegiate Cancer Foundation (NCCF)
(240) 515–6262
www.collegiatecancer.org
NCCF is committed to providing need-based financial support to young adult survivors who are pursuing higher education throughout their treatment and beyond. Furthermore, the Foundation promotes awareness and prevention of cancer within the young adult community.

National Organization for Rare Disorders (NORD)

(203) 744–0100

www.rarediseases.org

NORD's medication assistance programs help people with certain conditions. Check their website for a complete list of programs.

NeedyMeds

(800) 503–6897

www.needymeds.org

NeedyMeds is a free online clearinghouse to help people who cannot afford medicine or health care costs. This website includes information about services such as discount drug cards, Medicaid websites, federal poverty guidelines, and other useful information.

Nicki Leach Foundation

(904) 716–5394

www.nickileach.org

The primary mission of the Nicki Leach Foundation, a non-profit organization, is to provide modest financial assistance to young adults (eighteen to thirty) afflicted with cancer. Additionally, the foundation has an endowed scholarship fund at the University of North Florida.

Oligo Nation

www.oligonation.org

Oligo Nation is a community-driven, non-profit focused on advancing translational medical research on oligodendroglioma, a relatively rare form of brain tumor. Driven by the urgent need for new treatments, the organization reaches out to the roughly fifteen thousand families in America living with an oligo tumor.

Patient Access Network (PAN) Foundation
(866) 316–7263
www.panfoundation.org
PAN Foundation provides assistance to underinsured patients. Patients or a member of their medical team can apply online or over the phone; a determination for assistance is generally made within one business day.

Patient Advocate Foundation (PAF)
(800) 532–5274
www.patientadvocate.org
PAF offers information about financial resources and mediation services to assure access to care, maintenance of employment, and financial stability. Look for the Underinsured, Uninsured, and Financial Resource Directories, with information about alternative coverage options, as well as PAF's "Scholarships for Survivors" program.

Patient Advocate Foundation's Co-Pay Relief (CPR)
(866) 512–3861
www.copays.org
Insurance co-pay, co-insurance, and deductible assistance for cancer, genetic, and genomic testing.

Patient Services Incorporated (PSI)
(800) 366–7741
www.patientservicesinc.org

PSI helps people with specific conditions to pay their prescription copayments regardless of income. Check their website for a complete list of conditions. This list may change, depending on funding.

Ramps.Org
(847) 680–7700
www.ramps.org
Offers a national database of organizations across the country that help build accessibility ramps for those without the means to afford. Database contains charitable programs and institutions that offer both funding and building services.

RXAssist
www.rxassist.org/patients
Helps patients and caregivers learn about ways to use pharmaceutical company programs and other resources to help reduce medication costs.

RXHope
www.rxhope.com
Organization helps patients and caregivers navigate the system to obtain critically needed prescription medication and, at times, helps to get medication costs covered.

RX Outreach
(888) 796–1234
www.rxoutreach.org
Non-profit pharmacy whose mission is to provide affordable medications.

The Sam Fund
(617) 938–3484
thesamfund.org
Direct financial support and free online support and education for young adults.

Social Security Administration
(800) 772–1213
www.ssa.gov
Information on government disability and assistance programs.

SuperSibs!
(866) 333–1213
www.alexslemonade.org
Support for siblings of cancer patients via the Alex's Lemonade Stand Foundation.

Survivorship A-Z
www.survivorshipatoz.org/cancer
Survivorship A-Z is a web-based resource providing practical, legal, and financial information. The site includes the ability to make a computer-generated profile personalized to your legal, financial, and social situation.

Thrive Cancer Fertility Network (Central Texas)
www.thrivecancerfertility.org
(512) 535–4349
Provides financial help to young adults in Central Texas with fertility options in advance of cancer treatment, including support with retrieval, freezing, and banking.

Ulman Cancer Fund for Young Adults
(410) 964.0202
www.ulmanfund.org
A survivor-led organization based in Columbia, MD, with support and networking groups, college scholarships, a survival guide, and community grants to grassroots organizations.

United States Administration on Aging
(800) 677–1116
https://eldercare.acl.gov/Public/Index.aspx
Eldercare Locator connects you to services for older adults and their families.

United States Department of Health & Human Services
(877) 696–6775
www.hhs.gov
Information on public assistance and food stamps.

Vital Options International
(800) 518–2354
www.vitaloptions.org
Vital Options was founded in 1983 as the first psychosocial and advocacy organization for young adults with cancer. It also broadcasts The Group Room® cancer talk radio show weekly. They have expanded their mission to include direct support of patients, their caregivers and families across all chronic and life-threatening illnesses through the Selma Schimmel Vital Grant.

WellRX
(800) 407–8156
www.wellrx.com
Prescription discount card program.